The
Calcium Bomb

Also by Douglas Mulhall:

Our Molecular Future:
How Nanotechnology, Robotics,
Genetics, and Artificial Intelligence
Will Transform Our World

The
Calcium Bomb

The Nanobacteria Link to
Heart Disease & Cancer

Douglas Mulhall and Katja Hansen

Afterword by
Benedict S. Maniscalco, M.D., F.A.C.C.

THE WRITERS' COLLECTIVE   Cranston, Rhode Island

Independent Books for Independent Readers

ISBN 1-59411-101-4

Printed in the United States of America
10 9 8 7 6 5 4 3 2 1

Library of Congress Cataloging-in-Publication Data

Mulhall, Douglas.
 The calcium bomb / by Douglas Mulhall with Katja Hansen.
  p. cm.
Includes bibliographical references and index.
 ISBN 1-59411-101-4 (hardcover : alk. paper)
 1. Coronary heart disease–Etiology. 2. Coronary heart
disease–Treatment. 3. Coronary arteries–Infections. 4. Coronary
arteries–Calcification. I. Hansen, Katja, 1966- II. Title.
 RC685.C6M855 2005
 616.1'23–dc21
                                                2003008085

The Writers' Collective • Cranston, Rhode Island

For the billion or more whose lives

are affected by calcification.

Table of Contents

Disclaimer

This book examines the discovery of a potentially infectious trigger for calcification, as well as treatments aimed at reversing its impacts on the human body. The text is written in plain language. It is not intended as medical guidance and should not be substituted for a physician's advice. The authors based their work on information from patients, researchers, prescribing physicians, critics, and developers of the treatments. However, we the writers are not physicians. Treatments may have changed depending on when this book is being read. Questions about those treatments should be referred to a knowledgeable practitioner.

Many patients who have been treated for what seems to be a newly discovered infection are—according to their physicians—improving. On the other hand, studies of how quickly and consistently they improve have only just begun or have been recently published. Therefore, these are early days.

Despite this, we feel obliged to describe what is known now, and what still remains to be discovered, so that patients—especially those who have no other options—can ask their physicians and make decisions based on recommendations of those doctors. Individual conditions may or may not be addressed by such treatments. Everybody should seek qualified medical help prior to deciding for or against any therapy.

An Important Note on Definitions

Plain language is used in most of this book. An easy-to-read glossary is included to explain technical terms. Additionally, here is an introduction to terms used frequently throughout the text.

The term "calcification" is used here to describe abnormal calcium phosphate deposits in disease. The process is also known as "pathological calcification" and as "calcium deposits," but for convenience we usually use the short form. Calcification can also describe calcium deposits in geology, but the book does not focus on those.

Calcification is found often in "hardening of the arteries," which is the popular term applied to arteriosclerosis and atherosclerosis. In casual conversation, those names are often used interchangeably and can be confusing; so we explain the difference between them in the glossary. However, the important point is that many widespread conditions are associated with them, including aneurysm, calcified heart valves, congestive heart failure, enlargement of the heart, known as "cardiomegaly," heart attack, high blood pressure, stroke, and thrombosis (blood clots). Each has a calcification link.

Methods for measuring calcification have sometimes been given confusing acronyms, such as CT, EBCT, MRI, and IVUS. To simplify these, we often use the terms "scan" or "heart scan" in the text. Then we explain details in the glossary.

Particles known as "nanobacteria" have been discovered in disease-related calcification and have also been found in geological formations.

Nanobacterium sanguineum, "blood nanobacteria," and "human nano-bacteria" are terms used to describe the distinct type found in the human body. However, nanobacteria are still mysterious and may not be bacteria at all. They straddle the line between life and the chemical soup in which life is created. Due to conflicting views on what they are, they have been given an extraordinary variety of names, such as "agents," "artifacts," "bacteria-like life forms," "biofilm," "entities," "nanobes," "objects," "organisms," "particles," "pathogens," "self-replicating nanoparticles," "slime," and "vesicles." These terms have added to confusion over exactly what is being discussed.

This book touches on the controversy over what nanobacteria might be, but its main focus is on what harm they do to us and how to reverse their negative impacts.

Many chemicals and nutritional supplements are used to treat nano-bacteria. They are loosely referred to as "nanobiotics." They are not to be confused with drugs that work against other diseases at a very small scale and are sometimes also known as "nanobiotics." No one holds a monopoly on the name.

Part I
The Lit Fuse

One

You're on the Calcification List

Calcium is the stuff of life and of death. Every human must have it to survive. Yet, in many of us, a tiny fraction of it goes bad. This is known as "calcification." It is one of the most pervasive yet least understood medical conditions on Earth. Those who get it are often not aware of it until they suddenly become sick. For years, doctors had no solid evidence of where it comes from or how to get rid of it.

The good news: after more than a century of frustrating battles, the discovery of why calcium turns against us has led to new ways of protecting the body from this lifelong onslaught.

In plain terms, calcification is the hardening of our body tissue by calcium salts.[1] These salts contain other minerals, such as phosphorus, and are often toxic. They assault us when we are young, degrade us as we age, make us miserable, and then often kill us. Calcification is not normally a named disease, yet it is found in a range of illnesses. When the list is compiled, which is usually not done except for specialists, it is easy to see why such a menace escapes the limelight. Like a charlatan, it has many disguises (see fig. 1).

When doctors talk about this, they are not describing how the body uses calcium to build bones and teeth, but instead they are referring to a condition that attacks us constantly.

FOR WOMEN, A STEALTHY ENEMY

Breast and ovarian cancer strike fear into many women, while heart disease kills far more victims. Calcium deposits are found in each incurable condition. More women know about the deposits than before because

The Calcification List

- Aging of skin
- Alzheimer's (deterioration of brain function)
- Arthritis (osteo and rheumatoid)
- Autism (childhood brain disorder)
- Bone spurs
- Brain sand and brain cysts
- Breast implant calcification
- Bursitis (inflammation of the joints)
- Calcinosis cutis (calcium deposits in the skin)
- Cancer (bone, brain, breast, colon, prostate, and ovarian)
- Cataracts
- Deafness from middle ear ossification
- Diabetes (type 2 in adults)
- Gallstones
- Glaucoma (eye disease that degrades vision)
- Heart disease, notably arteriosclerosis and atherosclerosis
- Heterotopic ossification (bone formation in soft tissue)
- Hypoparathyroidism (low production of some hormones)
- Kidney stones, cysts, polycystic kidney disease (PKD)
- Liver cysts
- Macular degeneration (degradation of a part of the eyes)
- Ménière's disease (vertigo from inner ear malfunction)
- Multiple sclerosis (degradation of the nervous system)
- Parathyroid disease (affects hormones that balance calcium)
- Prostatitis (inflammation of the prostate gland)
- Psoriasis (inflammation of the skin)
- Salivary gland stones
- Scleroderma (hardening of the skin)
- Stroke (brain aneurysm and other blockages)
- Tendinitis (inflammation of the tendons)

Figure 1: *The calcification list. These conditions involve calcium deposits. See figure 3 for examples of where they occur in the human body.*

these show up on scans for heart disease and many cancers. Breast implant patients sometimes have to go back for surgery to remove calcium deposits that develop around the implant. These can be seen as distinct spots on mammograms and can be mistaken for possible cancer, resulting in additional surgery to test or remove the implant to distinguish the deposits from cancer. Calcified nodules or bumps may be felt under the skin around the implant.[2]

A less threatening but nonetheless debilitating affliction is arthritis, a general term given to joint diseases affecting a large minority of women and also men. Calcification is often found here. Many who have arthritis go on to develop heart disease, but the link has never been well understood.[3] Nor is the link understood between osteoporosis—the loss of calcium in the bones—and the seemingly contrary growth of calcium deposits that occasionally comes with it.

Lump these conditions together and you'll see that calcification is actively stalking most women.

That's not to say that the related illnesses are limited to females. Far from it. Men are afflicted just as frequently. However, until recently, with some of the most prevalent conditions such as heart disease, men have been more likely to be diagnosed. This is because for years women were given the mistaken impression that they were not as much at risk. Yet they were and are.

THREATENING SEX LIVES AND ASTRONAUTS

For those who worry about good looks and virility, calcification has nasty side effects. It gives the skin a hard sheen and feel, destroys elasticity, and contributes to ugly joint swelling. By restricting blood flow, it degrades a healthy appearance. In some men it forms painful lumps in the penis, making sexual intercourse unpleasant or excruciating, while in women it can do the same in the ovaries, causing painful experiences.

The process attacks astronauts who have been in space. The National Aeronautics and Space Administration (NASA) sees it as a serious health problem and a potential barrier to getting human beings to other planets. When astronauts go into space, and after they come home, they often are at risk of developing kidney stones, calcified coronary arteries, and arthritis "flareups." If, for example, stones disable them with agonizing pain, then space trips might have to be aborted.[4] Because of that, NASA tries to prevent this phenomenon. But success has been limited.

Calcification by Many Other Names

- Apatite (calcium phosphate)
- Atheromatous plaques (fibrous arterial plaques that in older persons often contain calcification)
- Biomineralization
- Brain sand (calcium deposits in the brain)
- Calcific
- Calcified deposits
- Calcinogenic (causing calcification)
- Calcium buildup
- Calcium deposition or calcium deposits
- Calcium phosphate (chemical symbol $CaPO_4$)
- Calcium salts
- Calculus (stone in the kidneys, gallbladder, etc.)
- Crystallization
- Cysts (many but not all cysts are calcified)
- Dystrophic calcification (hardening that results from disease occurring at the site of calcification)—this type occurs when calcium levels in the blood are normal
- Hard plaque (found in gums and arteries)
- "Hardening" of various bodily systems
- Hydroxyl apatite
- Metastatic calcification (results from disease occurring far from the site of calcification)
- Microcalcification (often found in breast cancer)
- Ossification (deposits of bone-like material in soft tissue)
- Plaque (soft and hard deposits in blood vessels)
- Spurs (as in bone spurs)
- Stones (such as kidney stones, gum stones, and gallstones)

Figure 2: *The many faces of calcification. These terms are used to describe calcification in disease. Each term depicts the same process; that is, formation of harmful calcium phosphate deposits in the body. Try these keywords in an Internet search engine. See figure 3 to learn where these deposits are found.*

What happens in space seems to be an acceleration of what happens to many of us here on Earth: calcium deposits show up in the wrong parts of the body.

STARS AND POLITICIANS HAVE IT

Being famous, young, or powerful does not get you off of the calcification hook. Everybody from rock stars to football players and politicians can have calcified tissue. Among the celebrities who've required operations to treat it have been leading network television show hosts, rock music icons, and at least one president of the United States. Hundreds of youthful sport figures have experienced calcification of their tendons and ligaments after sustaining injuries. Some never play again due to resulting stiffness and pain. Regardless of wealth or fame, calcification remains with them.

The rest of us are usually somewhere on the calcification list. If you're in your twenties or thirties, then it's possible that you've got calcified scar tissue from an injury. If you're over forty and have acute aches or pains repeatedly in your muscles or joints, then you've probably got calcification. For those who've been lucky enough to avoid injury or age-related calcification, some of your friends or relatives probably have the condition.

Even if you're not affected in those ways, then a good part of your income tax, sales tax, and health insurance premiums still goes to a medical system that struggles to treat diseases that are on the calcification list.

PAIN AND RELATIONSHIPS

Nothing is worse for our personal and work relationships than constant physical pain or the numbing drugs that we use to alleviate it. Together they irritate or disorient us and force us to act out of character, alienating those around us. Chronic pain can provoke relationship breakdowns by turning small misunderstandings into big ones or grinding us down day after day.

Many of these conditions are calcification related. Bursitis, tendinitis, arthritis, ovarian cysts, and spinal calcium deposits each require an army of painkillers, anti-inflammatories, and antidepressants to keep the throbbing to a dull roar. At a more serious level, calcification-related cancers and heart conditions bring on deep emotional and physical pain that is hard to quantify but plain to see and requires drugs that have unpleasant side effects. The term applied to these therapies that help us to get through the day is "pain management." As with the underlying conditions, we can

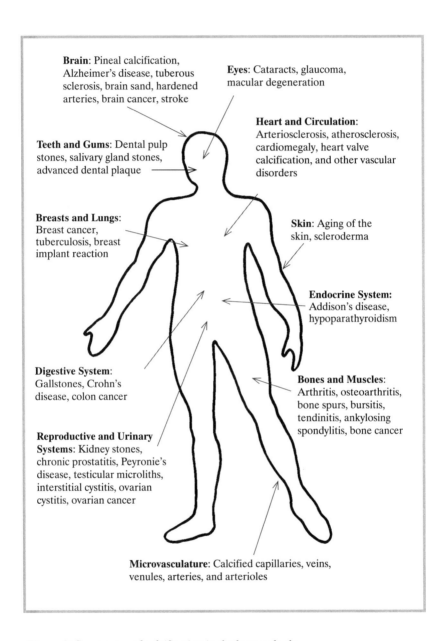

Brain: Pineal calcification, Alzheimer's disease, tuberous sclerosis, brain sand, hardened arteries, brain cancer, stroke

Eyes: Cataracts, glaucoma, macular degeneration

Heart and Circulation: Arteriosclerosis, atherosclerosis, cardiomegaly, heart valve calcification, and other vascular disorders

Teeth and Gums: Dental pulp stones, salivary gland stones, advanced dental plaque

Breasts and Lungs: Breast cancer, tuberculosis, breast implant reaction

Skin: Aging of the skin, scleroderma

Endocrine System: Addison's disease, hypoparathyroidism

Digestive System: Gallstones, Crohn's disease, colon cancer

Bones and Muscles: Arthritis, osteoarthritis, bone spurs, bursitis, tendinitis, ankylosing spondylitis, bone cancer

Reproductive and Urinary Systems: Kidney stones, chronic prostatitis, Peyronie's disease, testicular microliths, interstitial cystitis, ovarian cystitis, ovarian cancer

Microvasculature: Calcified capillaries, veins, venules, arteries, and arterioles

Figure 3: *Some areas of calcification in the human body*

manage pain but not get rid of it. While the cause goes untreated, stop-gap measures have ballooned into a vast industry.

Thus, calcified diseases not only disrupt our daily lives by jabbing at pain centers throughout the body, they also force us into a drug-and-treatment-dependent state.

KNOWN BY DOCTORS BUT NOT OFTEN DISCUSSED

Most patients have never heard of calcification because it hasn't been explained to them. This isn't surprising. Some of the terms used to describe it are very technical (see fig. 2).

But also, most doctors haven't known what triggers the condition or where it comes from, so they often don't pay much attention to it. Another frustration is that experts can't see much of the accompanying inflammation in arteries without using a risky invasive procedure.

The failure to cope with calcification has come partly from an inability to measure it. Fast scanning x-ray methods can show the big buildups. Terms such as "CT scan," "EBCT," and "ultrafast scan" describe progressive steps to let us see calcium deposits without cutting open the body. (See the glossary for definitions.) But these don't show the tiny particles. There has been no way to accurately test for such particles in blood.

FOOD AND FITNESS BOOKS MISS THE POINT

The idea that something in the body uses calcium to harm us is not explored in most diet and exercise books. Any mention of the mineral's downside usually concerns calcium deficiencies or overconsumption of supplements, not how our metabolism might abuse it.

Thousands of popular books touch on heart disease, arthritis, and cancer, but when it comes to calcification the descriptions are short. Understandably so. Most authors are hard pressed to explain the cause, pervasiveness, or effective treatment.

Renegade calcium is often found in joints that are damaged from overexercise or accidents, so you'd think that every nutrition and fitness book would mention it. But they don't. This is perplexing because many medical dictionaries cover such calcification.

AN ASTONISHING ARRAY OF ILLNESSES

Here are examples of calcification-related conditions, arranged by their presence in commonly known systems in the body. Some afflictions such as cancer and injuries occur throughout the body, so they are discussed in separate segments.

BRAIN

When calcium deposits block arteries and nerve endings in the brain, human thought processes are disrupted.

Alzheimer's disease. This illness destroys familiar personality traits. As the population lives longer, more victims are being afflicted. And it doesn't start only in old age.[5] Short-circuiting of synapses causes memory loss and confusion, progressing to violent outbursts and the inability to function. Calcium excesses are found in these synapses. Because too much calcium can lead to cell death, it is theorized that this overloads brain cells.[6]

Brain cancer. Calcium deposits are found in the craniums of brain cancer patients.[7]

Cranial calcification. Disorders other than cancer are associated with calcium deposits in the brain, sometimes known as "brain sand."[8]

Stroke. This is actually a "vascular" (circulatory) disease, but its main impact is on the brain. Hardening of the arteries throughout the body leads to clots that cut off the blood supply. This leads to catastrophic loss of memory, motor function, and reasoning power and then to death.

Multiple sclerosis (MS). Calcified plaques are found on the spine and in the brain of MS patients. Scientists say that a high prevalence of pineal calcification in MS suggests an association between MS and abnormalities of the pineal gland.[9]

Tuberous sclerosis. This disorder affecting newborns is caused by damage to genes that regulate cell growth. Its tumors affect the brain, skin, and kidneys. It is often associated with autism.[10] It is not to be confused with tuberculosis (TB).

BREASTS AND LUNGS

When certain diseases take hold, calcium deposits occur frequently in the chest cavity and breast tissue.

Breast cancer. It has been estimated that one in eight American women will develop breast cancer.[11] European and Japanese women are also at risk. The disease is a leading cause of death among females. Men can develop the same breast cancers that occur in women, although the percentage of men who develop them is much lower. A prime characteristic is calcified fibrous nodules.[12] The cause is unknown. Some treatments such as surgery, chemotherapy, and radiation can send breast cancer into remission.

Breast implant complications. Surgery is sometimes required to take out calcium deposits that form around breast implants.[13]

Tuberculosis. TB is a bacterial infection of the lungs, which still occurs in many developing nations. Calcified nodules are commonly found in tuberculosis patients.[14]

BONES AND MUSCLES

One of the great mysteries of medicine is why a calcium compound similar to the kind that forms bones also deforms them and gets into muscles or tendons to inhibit our mobility.

Arthritis. This affects tens of millions of Americans, Europeans, and Japanese, making it one of the most prevalent diseases in the industrialized world.[15] "Arthritis" is a general term applied to more than a hundred different types of joint problems, most of which are characterized by inflammation and painful movement, along with abnormal calcification in and around joints.[16] There are many therapies but no cure.

Bone spurs and bone cancer. Also known as "osteophytes," these are enlargements in the bony structure in the neck, back, and other weight-bearing or overused areas. Ligaments calcify, causing pressure on the spine and pain during movement.[17] Injections and surgical removal are the main therapies. Calcified bone spurs are also found in bone cancer.[18]

Bursitis and tendinitis. These are characterized by pain and stiffening of the joints, often accompanied by inflammation and calcification of the bursa and tendons.[19]

Osteoporosis. Loss of bone mass affects many women. There seems to be a link between this and calcification of the arteries. Calcium may go out of bones and into the arteries, but research on this is at an early stage.[20] Treatments include drugs and vitamin supplements, although these do not cure the condition.

EARS AND BALANCE

One cause of loss of balance as we get older is calcification, and in some cases it can also afflict younger persons.

Ménière's disease, vertigo. The inner ear regulates balance with fluid. Sometimes tiny stones in the ear seem to undergo a chemical change from calcium carbonate to calcium phosphate and then roll around in the fluid, leading to loss of balance.[21] The cause is unknown. There is no cure.

EYES

Glaucoma, cataracts, and macular degeneration are together responsible for most age-related vision loss among those over the age of fifty. Each is characterized by calcified buildups throughout the eye.

Cataracts. Calcified particles and fibrous tissue obscure vision in the lens of the eye.[22] They can usually be treated by surgically removing the lens, but are occasionally inoperable. Cataracts are also a good example of why there is a public perception problem with calcification. Many cataracts contain calcium deposits, but not much popular literature can be found that explains this.

Glaucoma. This causes the loss of a nerve fiber layer in the eye, leading to blindness. Millions are afflicted. Calcification is usually found at the site of the problem.[23]

Macular degeneration. The disease occurs in the central part of the retina, or "focus point" of the eye, causing decreased clarity and loss of central vision. Many older persons are affected.[24] Calcified nodules are often found in the membranes of the macula.[25] There is no known prevention or cure, although treatments are available for the initial stages.

DIGESTIVE SYSTEM

While we are taught that calcium is generally good for the digestive system, calcification certainly is not.

Colon cancer. One of the great killers, it often leads to other kinds of cancer. Calcified nodes are frequently found in a victim's colon.[26]

Crohn's disease. This inflammation in the intestinal tract can trigger secondary calcification-related complications, including arthritis, kidney stones, and gallstones.[27]

Gallstones. These have cores made of calcium carbonate or calcium phosphate.[28] Patients with gallstones can end up with liver disease due to obstruction of bile flow.[29] Calcification in the gallbladder can also be an indication of gallbladder cancer.[30]

GLANDS

When calcium deposits get into glands they can cause havoc with the tiny yet important amounts of hormones that those glands secrete.

Addison's disease. Calcification of the adrenal glands reduces hormone production.[31]

Hypoparathyroidism. This hormone deficiency causes abnormal use of calcium and phosphorus by the body. It is often characterized by kidney stones, cataracts in the eyes, and calcification in the brain.[32]

HEART AND CIRCULATION

Calcification is associated with acute coronary syndrome, aneurysms, angina, arrhythmia, arteriosclerosis, atherosclerosis, cardiomegaly (thickening of the heart muscle), circulatory problems, heart attacks, heart valve malfunction, high blood pressure (hypertension), stroke, and other vascular disorders. Treatments range from exercise and dietary changes to surgery and drug therapy. There are angioplasties (where a blocked artery is inflated for temporary relief) along with arterial stents (where a metal tube is put in the artery to keep it open). In bypass surgery, veins are taken from another part of the body and put around the heart to restore blood flow. But such therapies have a problem: calcification often contributes to blockages in stents and bypasses.[33] Many drugs are being developed to prevent such reblockage, but the cause is incompletely understood.

Diabetes. This disrupts the way the body works, resulting in thirst and increased urination. Diabetes is associated with obesity and atherosclerosis in adults, but it is also showing up at an alarming rate among children.[34] In diabetic patients, calcification is a strong predictor of death from heart failure.[35]

Calciphylaxis. This extremely fast and fatal form of calcification (death comes in one month) may occur in patients with severe kidney diseases and with a disease of the parathyroid gland—hypoparathyroidism.[36]

INJURIES

Everyone who has experienced a violent or repetitive stress injury to tendons and ligaments knows that the joint can stiffen afterward. This often results from calcification. Injuries from car accidents and falls can leave calcified tissue that stays with someone for life. When a joint is hurt, calcium deposits occur where scar tissue forms and blood flow is reduced. Plaque also collects where blood vessels bend or narrow naturally.[37] The cause is not known. Inflammation and calcification of joints can provoke acute pain and prevent movement. This is a serious problem for professional athletes and can get worse as they age, resulting in internal injury to arteries and in reduced blood flow.

SEX, REPRODUCTIVE, AND URINARY SYSTEMS

Calcification makes us less sexually attractive by degrading our appearance, but it also has more direct effects on our sex lives and on the body's capacity to excrete liquid waste.

Chronic prostatitis. This painful inflammation of the prostate gland is often accompanied by calcification.[38]

Interstitial cystitis. Chronic pain and spasm are usually associated with calcification and inflammation of the bladder wall.

Kidney stones. These often consist of cores of calcium carbonate or phosphate mineral.[39] Treatments include drugs, surgery, and diet, but there is no cure. Occurrence is on the rise.

Ovarian cysts, ovarian cancer, and fibroids. Painful calcified cysts in the ovaries may decrease a woman's ability to conceive children. Some cysts are benign. Others are cancerous.[40] Calcified fibroids often show up on radiographs of the pelvis. A benign tumor of the uterus is the most frequently diagnosed gynecologic tumor and occurs in a large minority of women older than thirty.[41]

Peyronie's disease. This type of calcification forms in the penis, causing it to be painfully crooked when erect and disrupting one's sex life.[42] Surgical removal of calcium deposits usually results in shortening of the penis. This is also associated with "erectile dysfunction," for which various virility drugs have been developed. There is no cure.

Testicular microliths. These are small, calcified stones in the testicles and are associated with cancer.[43]

SKIN

Calcification contributes to hardening of the skin. This is one of the most visible signs of aging.[44] Skin creams can disguise it but not reverse it.

Scleroderma. Here, inflammation and calcification lead to thickening, hardening, and tightening of skin, blood vessels, and organs. These can provoke heart, joint, and other problems. The cause is unknown, although it is associated with the overproduction of a fibrous protein in the body.[45] There is no cure.

TEETH AND GUMS

The mouth is seen increasingly as mirroring the condition of the body. This isn't surprising when we consider that most of what goes into us must pass through the mouth. As we'll see, there seems to be a link between calcified oral deposits and problems in arteries leading to the heart.

Dental calcification. It seems strange to say that calcium deposits are around our teeth, because most of us know that teeth are made of calcium. This type of pathological calcification occurs in the form of "calculus" near and beneath the gum line.[46] Equally serious are chronic inflammation and other types of calcification that develop in the gums and jaw, leading to tooth loss. Inflammation and clotting in tiny blood vessels around decayed teeth are remarkably similar to the clotting, or thrombosis, in heart attacks and strokes.[47] There appears to be a connection between calcification, inflammation, and clotting.

Salivary gland stones. These calcified stones are painful when they block glands that produce saliva.[48]

EVERYWHERE IN THE BODY: CANCER WARNING SIGNS

Calcium deposits are found frequently in cancer and are also a warning that malignancy may be about to erupt. Deposits in the brain, breast, colon, ovaries, gallbladder, and other areas are often cause for concern. Conversely, such deposits can trick medical experts by seeming to be cancerous when they are not, which at times results in unnecessary, risky surgery.

□

Collectively, these conditions bring us together in a perverse way by afflicting much of the population of the world. The epidemic is not limited to advanced industrialized economies. Its emotional and economic impacts are extraordinarily widespread.

Most of these illnesses have no cure. Treatments with anti-inflammatory medicines, steroids, narcotics, and surgery relieve the symptoms but usually not the cause.

Given that so many of us have calcification-related diseases, it makes sense to ask why educational literature pays such scant attention to calcium deposits and why few, if any, popular books are devoted to explaining them. Perhaps it's because researchers didn't know what triggers them or how to prevent them. Whatever the reasons, it's time to find out more—right now.

Two

When the Timer Starts Ticking

Despite the essential role that calcium plays in keeping us healthy, too much can harm us just as too little does.[1] An undersupply starves our cells, while a massive surplus can overload them. Therefore, the body strictly controls calcium levels with a sophisticated system that involves everything from bones to hormones and intestines.[2]

Strangely though, the calcification clock often starts to tick when calcium reserves in our blood are still balanced. You'd think that harmful deposits would form only when we have too much of the stuff, but that is often not the case. The mystery is, *why do we calcify when our calcium levels seem normal?*

This condition has a name: "dystrophic calcification."[3] And it happens a lot. Until recently, its origins were not understood.

Does it have to do with the calcium supplements that millions of us take? These are used by young and old alike to guard against real or perceived deficiencies. The supplements include vitamins that improve the body's ability to use calcium. Women often take these to protect themselves from bone loss. The Harvard School of Public Health reports that there is a scientific argument over how much good calcium supplements do.[4] Some authorities say they don't do much. Others say that we must increase our intake as we get older and that it is hard to take too much.[5] Furthermore, many experts state that calcium supplements have nothing whatsoever to do with calcification.

But the true mystery is that as we age we still often have sufficient calcium in us. Our bodies just don't use it in the same way as when we were

younger. We have a great contradiction. We stuff ourselves with supplements
while our bodies are often using calcium to build harmful deposits. That's
not to say that such supplements cause calcification, only that something
in the body misuses the mineral when levels seem fine.

Other studies show that calcification-related illnesses such as gallstones
and heart disease are connected to poor diet or lack of exercise. They also
show that the symptoms of such diseases can be reduced if we exercise
and eat the right foods (although as we'll see later there is disagreement
over what those foods are).[6] However, despite their undeniable benefits,
exercise and "eating right" do not seem to reverse the calcification.[7] Blood
vessels still get hard and calcium still seems to misbehave. Why is that?

THE GREAT CHEMICAL ACTIVIST

Calcium combines readily with other chemicals in ways that make calcification tough to get rid of.

Calcium was identified as an element long ago in 1808 and is known to
constitute roughly 3 percent of the earth's crust,[8] which makes it plentiful.
It joins with other chemicals in many compounds, including calcium salts,
or deposits, in the human body. These salts can be seen in victims who
have died from related diseases.

The main ingredient is a mix of calcium and phosphorus known as
"calcium phosphate." It is as hard as rock and can scratch some metal.[9]
Although it can be manufactured by living organisms, calcium phosphate
usually cannot be eliminated by antibiotics, other drugs, or radiation that
would make our bodies melt.

CALCIFICATION IS TOXIC

The impacts of calcification are described in well-known medical manu-
als.[10] These authoritative books show how the tiny particles that make up
calcified deposits can spark inflammation and changes in the rate of cell
reproduction.[11] Those are the hallmarks of infection and are sometimes
precursors to cancer. They point to a notorious yet often ignored trait of
such deposits: they can be toxic to human tissue.

That is why calcification is often referred to as being "pathological."
It is not the healthy process that feeds cells or builds bone but instead is
disease related.[12]

This nasty side is mystifying because calcium buildups are not always
toxic. Far from it. Calcium phosphate is used in a matrix to build our bones
and teeth. Here, we seem to have natural mechanisms that prevent the

compound from attacking the body. But mysteriously, some particles stray from these constructive paths to clog our joints, circulation, and organs. One researcher has cut through the scientific jargon by calling this "sand in our motor oil."[13]

When most experts describe calcium deposits, they play down the toxic effects. They portray the particles as just sitting around without doing much except gumming things up. Nothing could be further from the truth. Calcium phosphate particles are at the core of a process that attacks the human body. The assaults are continuous. They go on for as long as the deposits are in us.

START WITH THE TINIEST VESSELS

Something else lurks alongside calcification: microvascular disease. Up to forty billion capillaries supply the body with blood. Most of them are so small that blood cells squeeze through them one at a time. Without capillaries we would die because our cells would not get enough oxygen. Studies have found that capillaries expand and contract to control blood flow more than was known earlier, which makes their role paramount in keeping us healthy.[14]

As we age we feel less energetic because those capillaries harden, swell, and get blocked. At the early stage, swelling and irritation combine with a buildup of fats. When capillaries clog, the passages that deliver blood, nutrients, and oxygen are blocked. Corridors get more brittle year after year. Their inability to flex robs us of life-giving nourishment. This interferes with heart, liver, and other body tissues.

Calcification is part of the whole ugly process. It's insidious because we don't sense the onset. Many of us know the obvious symptoms from experiencing them or watching their impacts on others. Everything gets more difficult. It's tougher to work a full day in top form. We get out of breath more quickly. One day we feel a tightness that isn't supposed to be there. At this point blockages are advanced and body tissue has been damaged. Trouble usually follows.

WHAT'S THE CAUSE?

One of the more respected public medical sources, Harvard Medical School's Consumer Health information database, describes calcification in heart disease, optical nerve degeneration, erectile dysfunction, gum disease, breast cancer, and spinal cord pain.[15] Experts on the database who answer patients' questions state that there is no known effective way to get rid of calcified areas other than to surgically remove them (a procedure that is too risky in many situations and only a temporary fix in others), or just treat the symptoms.[16]

Experts agree on one other point: the cause of calcification is murky.[17] In the absence of a known mechanism, it has been relegated to the unexplained.

In this knowledge vacuum, billions of dollars are spent annually by patients, insurers, and governments so that doctors can prescribe medicines that let the body function while the underlying condition worsens. This helps to explain why treatments grow more expensive as time goes by. As symptoms multiply, it is increasingly hard to conceal effects on the body .

Some researchers suggest that these diseases are triggered by infection.[18] However, this is not reflected in explanations that are given to many patients.

Here's a test. Ask your physician what causes calcification. He or she might respond with something like "Calcification is caused by fatty deposits in the wall of the arteries."[19]

Then ask, "But how do those fatty buildups cause calcification?" Among the standard replies is this bit of techno-speak:

> [O]xygen free radicals create a chemical change (oxidation) in the bad cholesterol. In response, the immune system sends white blood cells to fight this new threat. Unfortunately, the result of the meeting between the white blood cells and the oxidized cholesterol is a fatty plaque that damages the walls of the arteries. These walls gradually narrow, and calcium deposits may collect in and harden areas where the walls are inflamed.[20]

In other words, fatty plaque somehow makes calcium salts "collect," then harden.

So, how are these calcium deposits collected? How do they get there? By what mechanism? How does this explain the calcium buildup in nonfatty tissues such as muscles and eyes?

The reply should be that there is no understood way for such fats to collect calcium salts.

Nonetheless, a standard response given to patients is that fatty deposits do collect these salts. Since fats and calcium salts come together in artery walls, fatty deposits must trigger calcification.

There are other standard answers aside from these, but they each have the same flaw: there is no proof. No clinical studies have shown that fatty deposits trigger calcification.

Regardless of that uncomfortable truth, the fatty deposit idea is the basis of treatments and low-fat diets for millions of patients. In many cases the treatments don't work or only slow the process instead of reversing it.

Most of us don't know about this dilemma because our doctors don't explain it. Professionals are familiar with calcium deposits, but they and the popular media often do not communicate that to patients—nor do consumer medical Web sites, where patients get much of their information. Although a World Wide Web search reveals more than one hundred thousand mentions of "calcification,"[21] often in reference to the human type, relatively few Web pages contain the term "cause of calcification."[22] Subscriber-based Web sites, usually reserved for experts, explore possible causes. Medical journals are also full of information about calcification but patients don't normally see these. While billions of dollars are spent researching why runaway minerals end up in the kidneys, gums, and arteries, most of the population is in the dark on this vital risk to human well-being.

MAKING IT WORSE

The frustration for radiologists is that the deposits stare at them from x-rays and other types of scans as white material, just as bones do, only in the wrong places—for example, in lines along the interior of heart valves, as stones inside kidneys, or as particles in the brain. Worse yet, many medical procedures cause trouble when used to treat these conditions. During open-heart surgery, heart-lung machines keep patients alive while the heart is shut down for repairs, but the brain can be damaged when capillaries collapse or are blocked, reducing oxygen supply.[23] Newer procedures reduce such risks but do not eliminate them.

Patients who have surgery to restore blood flow often experience renarrowing, or restenosis, due to inflammation and recalcification at the site where repairs were made.[24] Thousands of patients have stent reblockage each year and require more operations to reopen or replace them. Drug company researchers have discovered that stents block less if they contain time-released antibiotics or are radioactive.[25] But these don't stop the process in parts of blood vessels where stents were not inserted. (This reblockage problem is discussed further in chapter 10, where heart patients relay their personal experiences.)

Kidney stone and gallstone patients who have their stones pulverized by ultrasound also often experience recurrences. Sometimes the stones come back ferociously.[26]

The inflammatory devil

Prior to calcification becoming visible, a stealthier process generates blockages that harm us. Inflammation is the body's way of repairing injuries. This swelling comes when tiny capillaries expand to let infection-fighting cells pass through their walls to the point of invasion. Despite its benefits, inflammation can be dangerous. Just as swelling constricts parts of the throat when it is infected, a similar process can contribute to heart attacks when blood flow in large arteries is obstructed by inflamed vessel walls.

Studies also show a link between inflammation and cancer. Chronic inflammation is found alongside calcification in many cancers. But oddly, experts often do not draw the link between inflammation generated by calcium deposits and swelling at cancer sites, so the negative impacts are not well understood.

A fatal combination

After inflammation is triggered, an army of fats and fibrous deposits rush to the scene as part of the body's attempt to deal with the damage. These biochemical reactions are so numerous and complex that they confound medical professionals, let alone patients. However, what's important is that the interactions lead to development of "soft" and "hard" plaques. Most contain dead cell material that the body can't clear away (see fig. 4). Some plaques seem to be part of an attempt to fix injury to the artery.

Then there is another complication, sometimes referred to as a "ticking time bomb." This is clotting. In an injury, clotting helps to stop bleeding, but in already narrowed arteries, it can cause blockage that rapidly leads to death.[27]

Researchers have tried for years to understand the role of calcification in clotting, swelling, and plaque formation. These are usually found together, but no one has been able to show why.

Some experts say that calcification is part of a "walling off" process to control damage. It is a patch used, for example, in cysts that surround infections and cancers. This patching seems to occur after other processes, such as swelling, set the stage by attacking intruders.

However, that is a guess. There is no solid evidence that calcium phosphate is deliberately put there by the body as a patch. In fact, some researchers argue against this idea of calcification being used for healing.[28] They say that the body walls off injured areas including calcium deposits by surrounding the deposits with fibrous tissue. This suggests that calcification is the culprit and not the cure! The idea that the body tries to isolate

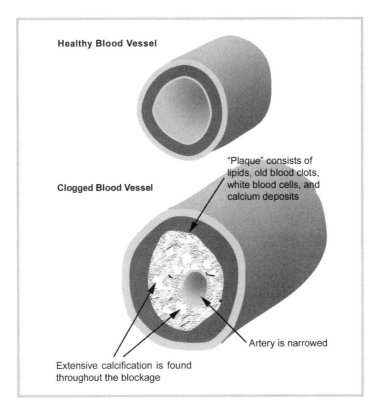

Figure 4: *The self-destructive process. Here are snapshots of the decades-long process that leads to blockage of blood vessels when the body responds to an invisible enemy. Top: Healthy blood vessel. Bottom: Formula for a heart attack or stroke. The advanced stages of cardiovascular disease. The process can start in childhood. Sometimes it will strike early, but usually it takes decades to accumulate critically.*

calcium mineral deposits due to their toxicity seems to make more sense than the idea that it uses a poisonous compound for repairs.[29]

The same researchers also argue that toxic calcification makes the defenses go into perpetual overdrive, attempting to wall off an enemy that won't go away. Why the body does this is perplexing because it doesn't do it with the calcium phosphate in our bones and teeth. If it did, then we'd be dead before we developed fully, as our immune systems attacked the material that forms our skeleton. Perhaps the immune system recognizes differences between pathological calcification and calcium phosphate that is in our bones. But how? Why?

Keep in mind that calcium is used, not just for bone and tooth manu-facturing, but also by every cell in the body for growing and dividing. That deepens the mystery. Why use toxic calcium salts to plug arteries that supply life-sustaining blood? It's a classic case of killing the whole to save a part. Oddly, the body seems to do it incessantly.

OUR TECHNOLOGY SEES ONLY SOME OF IT

Much of this blockage is hard to see. The soft tissue buildups, especially inflammation, are virtually invisible on conventional x-rays. They might show up if we let a machine trace the flow of radioactive dye through our arteries to see how much they are narrowed. But inflammation is still often obscured in such an angiogram.[30] The technologies are improving, yet they still don't let us see everything. Interpretations of these images are also prone to the subjective judgments of experts who examine them.

We see more when a physician shoves a catheter through our arteries with a camera attached, but such invasive tests are uncomfortable, risky, and expensive. Most of us don't agree to have them done, and doctors don't recommend them, until we have a problem. By then, the condition is seriously advanced.

At a smaller scale, virtually no technology is capable yet of mapping obstructions in the billions of capillaries that make up our microvascular system. The places where blockages begin go unexamined.

Together, these shortcomings suggest why about *half of those who suffer heart attacks show no prior symptoms*.[31] For them, doctors can't predict or see the real situation with regular detection technology.

Some of this problem may soon be solved with sophisticated scanners that let physicians see more soft tissue,[32] but these haven't yet helped the tens of millions who have blockages now.

▣

We've seen that calcification is a dangerous, furtive affliction that leads to no end of trouble. It is health enemy number one in many ways. So, what's the cause?

Three

The Nanobacteria Detectives

Scientists who make vaccines and other biological products are perplexed when cells that they use for experiments die mysteriously or stop growing although no contamination can be detected. In these cases, researchers have to throw out cell cultures and start again. This is expensive and poses a troubling possibility. The cultures might be contaminated with an unknown organism.

Much vaccine research depends on growing cells from mammals outside their bodies (in vitro). This involves fetal bovine serum, a blood product extracted from calf fetuses and used to help culture cells. The extraction is an ugly process that is opposed by animal rights groups, but researchers argue that vaccines produced this way have saved millions from polio and other diseases.[1] It is a loud dispute.

Because this serum comes from animals and the by-products are often transferred to humans, contamination of vaccines is a persistent worry. It affects whole populations. For example, polio vaccines were contaminated until at least 1963 with a virus that is thought to trigger some cancers.[2]

With such contamination in mind, Dr. E. Olavi Kajander (pronounced Kayander) found himself intrigued by the cell-death problem while working in 1985 as a postdoctoral research fellow in the laboratories of Professor Dennis Carson[3] at the Scripps Research Institute near San Diego, California.

This fascination would eventually lead Kajander to an astounding string of discoveries: A self-replicating particle so small that it confounded standard definitions for being "alive" was inhabiting farm animals and the human body. It was also triggering calcification that is tied to so many diseases.

WRONG TIME, PLACE, AND CONDITIONS

One project in Carson's department focused on improving human and mammalian cell culturing. Kajander, who holds a doctorate in biochemistry but was also trained as a medical doctor, began exploring why the cells died.

When he started his investigation, scientists already suspected that organisms might be present in "sterilized" cell culture media but could not be detected by routine methods. Earlier research by scientists at the Coriell Institute for Medical Research—among the largest human cell repositories in the world—suggested that slow-growing microorganisms might exist that escaped standard sterility testing because they did not replicate well under such conditions.

Around that same time, entities known as "mycoplasmas"—organisms without cell walls that are hard to detect—had been discovered. They also could not be cultured with standard techniques but were found to occasionally contaminate cell cultures. It had taken years to capture them due to this culturing problem.[4]

Kajander used that history to argue that other contaminants were evading detection. He guessed that researchers were attempting to culture them in the *wrong time frame, with the wrong types of culture media, and under the wrong conditions*. That was when the real detective story began.

To coax these organisms into the open, he began incubating cell cultures that were thought to be free of contamination. He did this in a nutrient-rich environment and for periods that exceeded normal incubation times.

This was not so revolutionary on its own because, for example, contaminants known as mycobacteria were also found to have long incubation periods. So in this way, Kajander was extending a field of investigation started by other scientists.

He soon discovered that something was growing. Its doubling time was extraordinarily long—ranging broadly from three to six days, compared to minutes, hours, or seconds for most bacteria and viruses. Because of this, it took weeks to develop a "biofilm colony" that was big enough to be detected. Organisms had been known to excrete such a slimy layer to protect and support themselves. The presence of the biofilm reinforced his hypothesis that an unusually extended incubation time was required.

The colony was not comprised of mycoplasma that can contaminate samples. This was important because some critics would later claim that Kajander had mistaken mycoplasma for these particles.

Looking through a microscope, he saw the first evidence of what would one day be known as "nanobacteria." Their presence was indicated by the biofilm that he'd been able to grow.

Where did they come from? Were they normally present in fetal bovine serum, or were his samples contaminated by accident?

The answers came two years later in 1987 after Kajander returned to Finland to establish his own cell culturing lab at the Biochemistry and Biotechnology Department of the University of Kuopio.

ANTICIPATING CONTAMINATION CRITICS

Finland may seem like a remote outpost to Americans, but many of its universities are known for solid interdisciplinary science. The University of Kuopio, dedicated to medical and biotechnology research, is one of those. A key to Kajander's nanobacteria discovery was the presence of the newest and best equipment, operated by competent experts, in a small university where he had easy access. A gamma irradiation facility was available for him to sterilize serum, medium, and equipment. This was to make sure that the contamination was not from the testing equipment or his methods.

After the serum was sterilized with high doses of radiation, the mysterious organisms would not grow in it. Then the organisms were reinjected into the sterile medium and were seen to be growing. This proved that the serum was not contaminated from an outside source.

That may seem like a trivial point, but contamination at such a small scale is a huge problem for researchers. It ruins many experiments. Kajander had to be certain that outside contamination was not the source. Proving this would be central to defending his discovery when it came under scrutiny years later.

THE CRUCIAL SUPPORTERS

He was lucky to be at Kuopio for other reasons. Succeeding heads of the university continued to support his work, although the potential for results remained uncertain for years. And while he himself had virtually no grant money to pay for his research, a professor of anatomy at the university had purchased what was then one of the best light microscopes in the world. Light microscopes are the traditional type that most of us see in high schools. They are not as powerful as the newer electron and atomic force microscopes, but the best ones can see down to the subcellular level. This let Kajander identify the tiny entities in his serum cultures. The vague term "entity" was applied to them because at that time he wasn't sure what they were.

Although the particles were each only about a hundred nanometers in size—too small to be seen individually by most light microscopes—their tendency to clump together in their biofilm made them visible under the powerful light microscope that he was using. They were also generating from their biofilm a semitransparent coating known as "apatite" (not appetite). This is a form of calcium phosphate mineral similar in some ways to that in bones. It made the particles much thicker—at least 200 nanometers in diameter—and far easier to see.

Oddly, electron microscopes that could see down to a smaller size didn't help at that stage. The rigorous processing required to prepare samples for viewing under such a microscope led to loss of the hard-to-cut particles. So their elusive nature confounded sophisticated detection instruments. Instead, the best of the "old-fashioned" light microscopes was used to make the first discovery.

In 1990 Kajander asked the Coriell Institute for Medical Research in New Jersey to help characterize the entities. It had been theorized that they were mycoplasmas discovered earlier by Coriell scientists, but after an investigation assisted by one of Kajander's students, it was concluded that they were not. Unfortunately, Kajander was also told that there was no funding for further investigation.[5]

Still, the acknowledgment by Coriell that something was there and that it was not mycoplasma gave Kajander ammunition to persuade the University of Kuopio to let him start a small repository to collect cell samples for experiments.

PATENTING NATURAL LIFE

He also launched a patent application for isolating and culturing what he was then calling a "nanobacterium." The full name of the genus and species that he'd found in human blood was *Nanobacterium sanguineum*, or "blood nanobacteria," which were also referred to later as "human nanobacteria." The patent was accepted in 1992.[6] Its terms were remarkably generous because they covered all methods for detecting nanobacteria and gave Kajander patented jurisdiction over what appeared to be a life form.

Scientists had been patenting genetic modifications to life (such as genetically altered mice) for some time, but until then few if any researchers had acquired a patent on a life form that occurred in nature. Olavi Kajander became one of the few individuals to patent what seems to be a naturally occurring life form, although there would soon be a hot discussion over whether nanobacteria qualified as being "alive."

This patent was awarded exclusively to Kajander. Neither his university nor a company was on the application. In an age of corporate and academic competition, it was extraordinary for such a basic discovery.

The patenting of nanobacteria was a profound step in science and law. It foreshadowed what has now become one of the great ethical debates of our time: who has the right to control life? Because the patent applies to what seems so far to be the smallest known form of life, it also suggests that someone might have legal domain over a submicroscopic universe that most researchers know absolutely nothing about.

However, as with other great discoveries—such as the description of DNA years earlier—few experts noticed when the patent was granted. Olavi Kajander slipped quietly into the record books—and into a mine field that would later jeopardize his career.

When he filed for the patent, Kajander also identified antibodies as diagnostic tools to test for nanobacteria's presence. Antibodies are like bloodhounds. They sniff out one type of organism and can be used to test for its presence among many others. This was a first step to finding it in samples and in the human body.

These new tools were crucial because conventional methods for identifying other organisms didn't work with nanobacteria and would lead other researchers to misidentify them.

THE FETAL BOVINE SERUM DISCOVERY

To learn more about them, Kajander had to find a good medium where nanobacteria could be cultured. Being strapped for funds, he tried the cheapest serum. This led to another discovery. When he compared the cheapest serum with the most expensive, he found more nanobacteria as contaminants in the cheap serum. The lower-cost product turned out to be a better source.

That source was fetal bovine serum from the United Kingdom, where fears over mad cow disease (also known as "BSE") had rendered the serum suspect, hence very inexpensive.

The British serum was full of nanobacteria. This discovery meant that fetal bovine serum from the United Kingdom was heavily contaminated. By extension, it suggested that *serum used for developing vaccines was also contaminated.*

For the next few years Kajander approached manufacturers of fetal bovine serum products and cell culture medium to tell them about the nanobacteria contamination in their serum. According to him, the companies agreed that there was a problem with the serum but said that they had no customers asking for nanobacteria-free fetal bovine serum culture media. There was no perceived risk. After all, what diseases did it cause? From a commercial viewpoint it wasn't worthwhile to pay for research into how the contaminants could be removed.[7]

For Kajander, it was another frustration. Companies whose products were contaminated acknowledged the fact, but didn't want to act.

This reluctance to investigate had also occurred earlier with mycoplasmas. They were discovered in the 1950s, but it was not until the 1980s that a demand arose for mycoplasma-free media.[8] Mycoplasma remains a problem today, causing illness among livestock and poultry.[9]

THE TURKISH MICROBIOLOGIST

By 1991, as Kajander was running out of time and money, one of life's great coincidences transformed his isolated search for the keys to nanobacteria. One day as he was walking the corridor of his laboratory, the departmental secretary stopped him to ask what she should do with an application from a postdoctoral microbiologist.

Kajander couldn't believe his luck. A day earlier, he had received a response from the National Institutes of Health (NIH) in the United States telling him that if he wanted to have a grant to explore nanobacteria, he'd have to find a qualified microbiologist. He immediately contacted the applicant, Dr. Neva Çiftçioğlu, who was based in Turkey.

In a telephone interview, Kajander sensed her enthusiastic tenacity and hired her forthwith. He lacked the funds to pay her, so the work would have to depend on her scholarships. In fact, by the time Çiftçioğlu arrived, Kajander had temporarily abandoned his experiments on nanobacteria due to financial constraints. But after examining the work that he had done, she was intrigued and continued with the research.

Çiftçioğlu would prove to be the missing link in Kajander's quest. Until then, microbiological skills such as hers had not been applied to basic nanobacteria research. Like Kajander, she was experienced in medical investigations and had a deep concern for what made patients sick. Kajander the biochemist and Çiftçioğlu the microbiologist began to produce results.

The first of many crucial steps that Çiftçioğlu took was to develop special staining methods that would let the nanobacteria be seen and studied more easily. By the end of 1991 she'd succeeded in doing this routinely.

In the ensuing years, Çiftçioğlu contributed significantly to the original discovery of Kajander's nanobacteria by slashing the time it took to culture them and by developing antibody methods to detect them in living mammals. It would not have been possible to find or measure a treatment's effectiveness for nanobacteria without such discoveries. They were so compelling that the U.S. National Aeronautics and Space Administration later put Çiftçioğlu at the head of its program to investigate whether nanobacteria were the cause of calcium deposits going haywire in astronauts.

Development of these methods also led to the eventual founding by Kajander and Çiftçioğlu of a Finnish company, Nanobac Oy, which offered nanobacteria-related analytical services. This was the first commercial step for nanobacteria research while work continued at the university.

THE ACCIDENTAL CONTAMINATION

Accidental contamination often ruins experiments, but also plays a defining role in discovery. Contamination led researchers to discover penicillin many decades ago when mold was found to be growing in a petri dish. A similar accident catalyzed nanobacteria research.

One day Çiftçioğlu confessed to Kajander that she had accidentally contaminated some samples. Kajander was about to scold her because from the start he'd warned her against the risk of contamination. However, she was quick to add that it produced a surprising result. The contamination had shown that nanobacteria had "eaten" the by-products of the corrupting bacteria as food. It appeared to be a sort of symbiotic process. This discovery let the scientists culture nanobacteria more quickly.[10] It also suggested how the organisms survive and flourish.

"STERILE" BLOOD?

The clues to how nanobacteria might feed on organisms pointed to why scientists had missed them for so long. Nanobacteria required a complex environment in which to develop. That environment was present in human urine and blood—which years earlier had been thought by doctors to be normally "sterile," i.e., free of living contaminants in healthy humans.

Older physicians may remember that from the day they entered medical school, they were told that healthy blood was a normally sterile environment. If it was not—the reasoning went—then we'd probably die because we'd be battling constantly against infection in our blood, suffering self-destruction provoked by our immune system as it turned on the body.

Furthermore, the mistaken idea that had led to blood transfusion-related disease was that if a contaminant could not be grown from blood by using standard culturing and detection techniques, then the blood was sterile.

The discovery that nanobacteria survived well in blood was part of a multidecade string of revelations that blood was not a normally sterile environment. Pathogens such as *Bartonella* and *Brucella* had also been found to inhabit blood.[11] In that context, the idea that nanobacteria were able to roam the circulatory system for years was not so special or surprising.

However, Çiftçioğlu and Kajander's finding supported the added idea that an internal battle was being waged at a rate so slow that it was hard to discern with the most advanced techniques.

HOW DID SO MANY SCIENTISTS MISS IT?

Other evidence suggested that the nanobacterial world has more than just one lifelike form. As we'll see later, it may contain many undescribed forms that are vast in numbers, magnificent in their internal mysteries, and far more ancient than *Homo sapiens*.

Researchers have only begun to discover this universe. Why? The short answer is, they were looking at part of it but didn't see it.

A glance at the authoritative *Merck Manual of Diagnosis and Therapy*, used by thousands of doctors, shows how clear the signs of nanobacteria have been. In its description of basic calcium phosphate disorders, the manual explains that "crystals occur in snowball-like clumps in rheumatic conditions."[12] The term "snowball-like clumps" is noteworthy because it describes the same clumps of the same crystals that characterize calcium-coated nanobacteria.

While researchers had the tools to see them, they didn't recognize them because the diagnostic methods to isolate and identify the nanobacteria component were missing. As we'll see, classical diagnostic methods gave abnormal readings or failed to identify key characteristics.

Kajander and Çiftçioğlu argue that some features of nanobacteria make it clear why researchers had gazed at them daily without knowing what they were:

- ▣ They form a calcium phosphate shell that makes them look like a lump of rock instead of something that's alive.

- ▣ They are hard to isolate with conventional diagnostic tools because they grow at a slow rate and seem to have a unique genetic structure.

◙   They lurk in the twilight zone between life and the chemical
    processes that spark life.

It is hard to imagine that nanobacteria were overlooked in an age when most of the plentiful things on Earth seem to have been discovered. But the failure to identify plentiful substances is not new. A good example occurred in physics with subatomic *neutrinos*, which are now recognized as being among the most abundant substances in the universe. Although their existence was postulated in mathematics in the 1930s, they could not be detected for decades because physicists didn't have the diagnostic tools. Nonetheless, trillions of neutrinos were passing through every human being, and everything else, each millisecond of every day.[13]

OVERCOMING THE BARRIERS TO DETECTION

Although nanobacteria had been found in fetal bovine serum as early as 1985, it took until the mid-1990s to find them in disease. The delay was due partially to the cost and time to develop "monoclonal antibodies" that are used for finding infections in the human body. The two scientists had to develop such methods themselves, with virtually no outside money. Often they had to use their own personal savings to pay for the research, sometimes for more than a year at a time. The funding problem would continue to dog their investigations despite later involvement of renowned research institutions and corporate investors.

Here are some of the technical barriers that made the job so tough:

Nanobacteria in their mature calcified form may be seen with a very good conventional light microscope if they are in clusters or biofilm. However, it's what's beneath their shell that is mysterious. Finding that requires far more powerful tools. The trouble is, preparing samples for a transmission electron microscope often results in loss of nanobacteria because they are so hard to slice into sections for examination. Their small size and special structure confound conventional preparation methods.

One of Neva Çiftçioğlu's challenges was to overcome these detection barriers in the human body. She started by screening kidney stones and dental plaque for nanobacteria. This could be done only after antibodies were developed to do the tests. It was time-consuming, took up lab resources, and cost money.

She also had to deal with the special structure of nanobacteria. Their genetic strands seem unique. The precise gene sequence is hard to detect because chemicals used to strip off the calcium shell may also disrupt the nanobacteria's genetic structure. Regular gene sequencing methods therefore had to be modified.

It was hard to culture and isolate nanobacteria because they replicate very slowly—over three to six days to produce a daughter cell instead of just minutes or seconds for many bacteria and viruses.[14]

One more barrier stopped researchers. Few dreamed that a self-replicating particle could be as small as 50 to 200 nanometers in diameter (see fig. 5) or that such a tiny thing could generate a calcified coating. Other lifelike particles such as viruses can be that small, but they cannot replicate without depending on other life forms to help them, and most do not form calcium coatings.

By eventually overcoming these barriers to detection, Çiftçioğlu and Kajander together pried open the doors to the nanobacterial world.

WHAT GETS RID OF NANOBACTERIA

First they had to optimize ways of stripping off the apatite coating to get at proteins in the nanobacteria. Those proteins were essential for determining the particles' characteristics. This part of the research led the scientists to what could be seen as a great medical discovery. They found that tetracycline and other chemicals such as bisphosphonates eliminate the "naked" organisms once their calcium coating has been dissolved. In so doing, they invented what would be the basis for a formula to treat nanobacteria infections: *dissolve the protective calcium layer, then eradicate the underlying organism.*[15]

By 1998, they had applied for a patent, which was subsequently granted by European and American patent authorities and now forms the basis for treatment.

While these discoveries were unfolding, Kajander and Çiftçioğlu sent out the first of many papers that were to be rejected by scientific journals whose editors didn't believe nanobacteria could exist or who demanded expensive and lengthy reverification. Such rejections are not unusual. The works of many renowned discoverers, including Nobel Prize winners, have been rejected by publications early in those researchers' careers for similar reasons. It was part of a grueling initiation that Kajander and Çiftçioğlu had to get used to, especially because they were rewriting the book on what it is to be "alive."

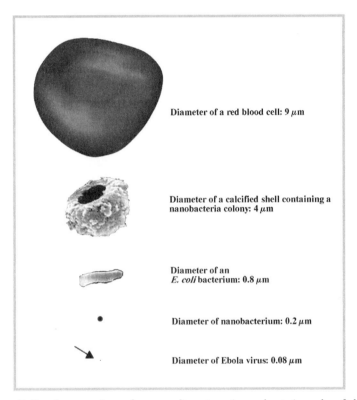

Diameter of a red blood cell: 9 μm

Diameter of a calcified shell containing a nanobacteria colony: 4 μm

Diameter of an E. coli bacterium: 0.8 μm

Diameter of nanobacterium: 0.2 μm

Diameter of Ebola virus: 0.08 μm

Figure 5: *Rough comparison of average diameters. A nanobacterium, dwarfed by a red blood cell, is far smaller than a commonly known bacterium but larger than many viruses. Calcified shell contains many nanobacteria.*

Four

Challenging the Definition of Life

S cientists stunned the world some time ago with a claim that "cold fusion" could occur in a test tube. The prospect of limitless cheap energy sparked excitement worldwide, but this dissolved quickly as other researchers reported that they could not duplicate the results.[1]

Some critics have also said that nanobacteria are the cold fusion of microbiology and have made their opinions known broadly.[2]

Is the comparison legitimate? Contrary to cold fusion research, the detection and description of human nanobacteria were by no means one-off experiments that couldn't be replicated. Instead, the journey began with discovery of the particles themselves, then progressed to methods for staining them, culturing them, finding them in other media such as vaccines, growing them in lab animals, then isolating them in kidney stones and heart disease. Most early discoveries were made by a team in Finland under the leadership of Kajander and Çiftçioğlu. That soon expanded to a wider group. Detection of nanobacteria in heart disease was first recorded by one of their collaborators, László Puskás, at the Hungarian Academy of Sciences.[3] His results were later repeated by scientists at America's Mayo Clinic and at the Austin Heart Center at the University of Texas.[4] Other scientists at the University of Illinois School of Medicine detected nanobacteria in kidney disease.[5] So did researchers at the Postgraduate Institute of Medical Education and Research in Chandigarha, India.[6] Signs of the infection were also discovered in ovarian cancer[7] and in the heart valve of a patient with end-stage diabetes.[8]

COULD SO MANY BE WRONG?

Despite such discoveries at reputable research institutes, was it still possible that nanobacteria didn't exist, that they were mistaken for something else, and that this was at best a cold fusion–type error or at worst a hoax?

That's what some critics claimed. However, the very basis for the argument testified to how masterful nanobacteria were at deception. Due to a tiny size and special structure, the particles confounded the preconception of what is "alive" and the definition for "bacterium." Furthermore, due to their name they got mixed up in arguments over everything from Martians to particles in ancient Earth rocks.

> The idea of the existence of nannobacteria [sic] has been greeted with howls of disbelief by the majority of the biological community, who contend that these minute bodies cannot be bacteria because they are too small to contain the necessary genetic machinery for life.[9]

So wrote Dr. Robert Folk, the discoverer of geologically based particles that he named "nannobacteria" (with two *n*'s).[10] His passage summarizes some of the first shots fired at him and other researchers in the fight over whether these tiny entities exist or are "alive."

Folk is credited with being the first to identify nanoscale organisms in geological rock specimens from hot springs. It is said that he did this around 1986, although he didn't publish his findings until many years later.

As it turns out, the particles found by Folk may be distinct from human nanobacteria. His may be bacteria and the others not. Nonetheless, in both cases, the question at the time was, are they too small to be alive?

ENTER THE MARTIANS

The image confusion accelerated in 1996 when one of NASA's chief scientists, David McKay, stunned the space exploration community by publishing a paper stating that tiny fossils named "nanobacteria" had been discovered in a meteorite that apparently came from Mars and had been found in Antarctica.[11] This garnered wide publicity as claims and counterclaims flew over what had been discovered and whether the entities resulted from contamination of samples. Were they just inorganic "artifacts" instead of once-living organisms? The controversy over "Martian life" lent a surreal quality to the nanobacteria discussion. For example, one news article about it was entitled "The Martians in Your Kidneys."[12]

TRANSFORMING THE LIFE-SEEKING PARADIGM?

Around the same time, geologists led by Dr. Philippa Uwins discovered what appeared to be a similar organism in Australia:

> We refer to these features as nano-organisms or nanobes to indicate their significant difference in size to Eubacteria and Archaeae . . . Our thesis is that nanobes are biological organisms.[13]

Their next discovery was DNA markers in nanobes.[14] That added another spark to the controversy. Did these lifelike characteristics come from contamination of samples instead of from the particles themselves? Some said yes.

However, at least one further development supported Uwins. In 2002 a team led by Professor Karl Stetter of the University of Regensburg, Germany, discovered a nanoscale organism in volcanic vents and named it *Nanoarchaeum equitans*.[15] The team later published that they had sequenced the particle's genome.[16] They had also found that one of the small subunit ribosomal RNA genes of *N. equitans* had different characteristics from what had been known until then. Therefore, traditional methods for identifying it did not work. For years, scientists had depended on certain standard testing procedures as proof of life. The discovery about *Nanoarchaeae* suggested that these tests alone were insufficient for uncovering lifelike processes. It also suggested that a subuniverse of so-far undetected nano-organisms might be in the environment.

Was this proof that entities such as human nanobacteria also existed? On its own, no. However, it did show that if only conventional means were used to look for nucleic acids in such tiny organisms, researchers might wrongly conclude that they were not alive. Worse yet, investigators might miss them altogether.

At stake in the scientific community was no less than how to look for the origins of life on Earth and possibly other planets. Whoever got their ideas accepted about tracking down nucleic acids might set the standard for finding novel life forms. If, for example, nano-organisms were shown to exist but not to be detectable with standard testing, then this might alter the life-seeking paradigm.

Someone who could prove this would be eligible for a lot of research funding, so the argument over how to look for novel life wasn't just about theory. It was about money. This virtually guaranteed that the discussion would be a contentious one.

Thus, components of life were popping up in nanoscale entities that didn't seem to resemble other types of life: in Australian samples, Icelandic samples, and in human nanobacteria that trigger disease.

Nano-organisms in geology were important because they suggested that the smallest known living thing existed in large numbers. But so far it had no known genetic link with Kajander and Çiftçioğlu's human nanobacteria. First results from genetic tests suggested that the link between nano-organisms found in geological formations and human nanobacteria was tenuous because *Nanoarchaeae* were distinct from human nanobacteria.

This was not a bad thing. It only suggested that nano-organic families are diverse—perhaps greatly so.

However, none of that was known in the late 1990s when information about human nanobacteria was being published from conferences where "Martian" nanobacteria were also discussed. Therefore, media confusion between rock-based and human nanobacteria accelerated.

This "guilt by association" cast new attention on Kajander and Çiftçioğlu's work. Due to the small size of these Martian and human nanoparticles, the International Society for Optical Engineering took an interest in both. By 1999 numerous papers by Kajander and Çiftçioğlu about human nanobacteria had been published by the society. Thus, a connection with another planet provided an opening to publish.

That connection was a double-edged sword because the Martian meteorite hypothesis had been attacked as nonsense, and the Optical Engineering Society's journal was not regarded by biological scientists as an authoritative source.

Early skepticism had partially been dispelled when Kajander's respected mentor at Scripps in California, Professor Dennis Carson, published an article in *Proceedings of the National Academy of Sciences* in 1998, concluding that nanobacteria were a cause of pathological calcification in humans.[17] This foreshadowed what would come years later in 2004, when a leading peer-reviewed journal specializing in kidney stone research published results confirming that human nanobacteria had been found in kidney stone patients and had been cultured. The paper concluded that sufficient proof had been found to show that these nanobacteria were alive.[18] Also in 2004, a research group in Charleston, West Virginia published findings of nanobacteria in the heart valve calcification of an end-stage diabetes patient.[19]

Still, some scientists and doctors claimed that nanobacteria didn't exist or weren't alive. The "cold fusion" analogy persisted despite so many new findings.

A striking side effect of such attacks was to slow research into whether nanobacterial infections existed or what treatments might be used. Perversely, instead of sparking efforts to prove or disprove earlier findings, the criticisms seem to have led some American institutions *not* to investigate.

Let's examine the arguments to see if they merited such a response.

THE POSSIBILITIES

Human nanobacteria have been defined by their discoverers as nanometer-scale entities that self-replicate and manufacture carbonate apatite structures (calcium phosphate mineral).[20] For a description of what are claimed to be steps in the life cycle of nanobacteria, see figure 6.

Here are some of the main possibilities put forward by proponents and critics about the existence of human and other types of nanobacteria:

◙ Possibility A: They are alive, perhaps in some way that scientists do not understand. Various self-replicating particles of nanometer scale have been found by scientists in hundreds of samples from meteors, volcanoes, geological core samples, vaccines, and from the blood of human patients. Some of these particles manufacture nucleic acid or have had their genes mapped. They seem to be previously undiscovered forms of life, although they have not yet been shown to be related to each other.

◙ Possibility B: Mistaken life signs. All findings resulted from experiments contaminated with DNA or RNA. Alternatively, scientists found nonliving crystals that attract DNA and replicate without being alive.

◙ Possibility C: It's all a hoax. The scientists who purported to make the original discoveries used fraudulent claims to pull the wool over the eyes of many reputable institutions, despite results being replicated by several independent teams.

Given the breadth of evidence, it is certain that scientists have found *something*. However, these "somethings" may each be dramatically different. Human nanobacteria and geological "nannobacteria" are probably not the same, but both have DNA and RNA fragments tied with life processes. Human nanobacteria have been found often in the human body and show definite signs of being infectious.

Critics claim that a self-replicating crystalline structure—in other words a rock that grows chemically—could exhibit or cause each of these

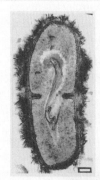
According to its discover-
ers this is a nanobacterium
250 billionths of a meter
thick. Note the "hairy" apatite
layer around the exterior.
This is solidifying calcium
phosphate.

(Bar in picture = 100 nm)

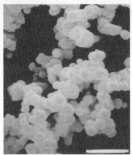
A colony of nanobacteria hang-
ing together with biofilm. It takes
weeks or months for one nanobacterium to replicate enough times
to produce such a colony.

(Bar = 1 μm = 1000 nm)

A group of nanobacteria beginning to congregate and form a calcified shell that will contain the colony
[picture taken after a three-month
culturing period].

(Bar = 200 nm)

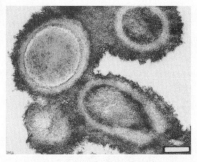

Figure 6: *Nanobacteria and calcification. Photos are copyright (1998) National Academy of Sciences, U.S.A.* [Source: E. Olavi Kajander and Neva Çiftçioğlu, "Nano-bacteria: An Alternative Mechanism for Pathogenic Intra- and Extracellular Calcification and Stone Formation," *Proceedings of the National Academy of Sciences USA* 95, no. 14 (1998): 8274–79.]

characteristics. It could also accidentally contain DNA captured from living material. Yet such a crystal is not alive.[21]

Defenders have shot back that DNA capture and transfer by crystals do occur,[22] but this does not explain why RNA synthesis has been observed with nanobacteria,[23] and it certainly does not explain how the genes of *Nanoarchaeum equitans* could have been sequenced. No crystal can manu-facture a full set of genes.

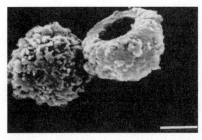

Scientists have been aware of these igloo-like structures for decades. They often are found at the centers of kidney stones. The structures here were grown outside the human body without serum. This simulates conditions in the human body when nanobacteria have been cut off from nutrients by the body's defensive response. Under those conditions they seem to increase biofilm production, congregate, and form shells. The flat side of the igloo where the hole is located marks where the shells were attached to the petri dish. (Bar = 1 μm)

The beginning of a war? Nanobacteria attacking healthy cells. By infiltrating cells, nanobacteria get energy and resources to replicate. They also seem to trigger an immune response that results in inflammation and dangerous deposits.

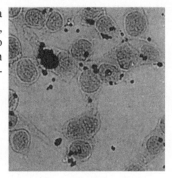

Figure 6 *(continued): Sequence and accompanying captions have been composed by the authors based on discussions with Çiftçioğlu and Kajander.*

Because of this, proponents accuse critics of stuffing nanobacteria into a familiar box instead of acknowledging such special traits and establishing a new category of organism.[24]

Other critics bring up the *C* word: contamination of samples. It has been said that DNA from other sources is what all these scientists are finding. Contamination is nothing new, and it is a big problem at this small scale. However, it can be misused as a convenient explanation when die-hard opponents run out of other arguments. Without other proof that contamination occurred, it has to be taken with a grain of salt.

Still other scientists argue that the smallest possible size for a free living, DNA-based organism is a diameter in the size range of 200 to 250 nanometers.[25] Anything smaller, they argue, cannot contain the types of DNA and other materials required for something to be "alive" by commonly accepted definitions. Nanobacteria have been identified in the 50–300 nanometer range, putting some of them near or below that minimum size.

But the key word is "some." Nanobacteria larger than 200 nanometers have also been found and meet the size criterion. Furthermore, scientists including Mayo Clinic researchers and Kajander and Çiftçioğlu have said that supporting evidence of nucleic acids coming from the interior of human nanobacteria has been observed.

Regarding the smaller particles, Kajander himself has pointed out that these may not be complete nanobacteria but rather "buds," or fragments, from larger mature nanobacteria.[26] He is one of the first to say that these smaller fragments may not themselves be "alive" in the conventionally accepted sense. He adds that nanobacteria may force us to redefine what is "alive," due to their special structures.

Normally people think that a living entity is a cell—that it is surrounded by a membrane and that it exists in a closed compartment. Now there is a possibility that nanobacteria may consist of basic units that on their own are so tiny that they have to come together to make a living organism.[27] Some observers speculate that before they assemble into larger units, these smaller units may rely on a host organism to survive.[28]

Kajander further cites arguments by some scientists that the smallest living thing is a single gene—something far smaller than a cell—and that genes come together to form larger living entities.[29] That, he says, also challenges the definition of living organisms.

When does a primordial thing containing complex chemicals and genes—and exhibiting lifelike behavior—become alive? DNA tests suggest that nanobacteria are alive but are different types of organisms because they do not respond to the standard form of DNA testing.

Do nanobacteria have some lifelike characteristics but lack others so they are in a special category? Viruses and prions have their own categories, but whether they live or not is still debated. Why not accept the same ambivalence for nanobacteria?

This takes us back to the "bacteria" part of the name. The discoverer laments that this leads scientists to compare them with bacteria such as *E. coli* found in the intestines, which are larger and have a different structure.[30] It seems strange that scientific investigation might be misdirected or misinterpreted due to a name, but in this case the association with bacteria and everything that they entailed was causing just such confusion. It triggered debates over bacterial characteristics in a situation where they were not expected to be found. It provoked media misunderstandings that required constant correcting.

THE UGLY PARTS

The argument got nasty in 1999 when the journal *Nature* published an article reporting that a group of academics in Finland had accused nanobacteria discoverer Kajander of unethically overstating results of his research. No one was more surprised than Kajander himself, who first read about it in that journal. The accusation came from someone who apparently had done no lab research of his own on the organism. Still, one journalist approached the story this way:

> Over the past few years, a group of Finnish scientists have expressed concern that Olavi Kajander has failed to produce the necessary biochemical evidence to prove that the particles he claims to be nanobacteria are in fact alive. Kajander says that he has shown this, and he has supporters of his own, including some prominent researchers at the US space agency NASA.[31]

After a formal investigation, the University of Kuopio's Ethics Committee—the group that the complaint was filed with—concluded in 2000 that:

> [i]n the view of the Research Ethics Committee this is a matter of scientific dispute and not of misconduct or fraud in science.

> The Rector has examined the documents and the data presented and has concluded that the request for investigation by Jouni Issakainen, [M.Sc.], warrants no further actions by the Rector . . . The complaint . . . against Docent [full professor], research director Olavi Kajander, Ph.D. is herewith rejected.[32]

So, the complaint was thrown out as unfounded—not once but twice, when a central scientific ethics committee of Finland also rejected it.[33]

Unfortunately, news of Kajander's vindication couldn't reverse the damaging delay to some of his work. His exoneration also went unreported in the journal *Nature*, where the original story had run. This shows how the mere news of an accusation can set back research, especially if science media don't cover the outcome of an official investigation after the charges have already been reported.

The controversy escalated when an American researcher, John O. Cisar, using a grant from the U.S. National Institutes of Health, wrote a paper with other scientists explaining that they had only partially replicated Kajander's results. They were able to culture the entities and take electron microscope photographs of them but were unable to identify that they contained DNA unique to that life form. The Cisar team concluded that these data do not provide plausible support for the existence of a previously undiscovered bacterial genus. Instead, we provide evidence that biomineralization previously attributed to nanobacteria may be initiated by nonliving macromolecules and transferred on "subculture" by self-propagating microcrystalline apatite.[34]

In other words, although the researchers were able to culture them and photograph them, these entities could not be bacteria and were not alive because the experiment hadn't managed to characterize them as such.

A DECISION NOT TO INVESTIGATE

On the basis of an interpretation of that finding, an arm of the U.S. Food and Drug Administration (FDA) concluded that nanobacteria don't exist and therefore are not potential contaminants in vaccines.

The absence of the FDA and the U.S. Centers for Disease Control and Prevention (CDC) from investigations into nanobacteria in human and animal disease was one of the stumbling blocks to research. It was especially perplexing in view of the pervasiveness of calcification in disease and the inability of most FDA-approved drugs to touch calcium deposits. It was more mystifying because another influential U.S. government agency, NASA, was investigating nanobacteria as a potential health problem in astronauts.

Here is how the FDA advisory group decision not to investigate nanobacteria seems to have been reached:

In November 2002, as part of their regular quarterly meeting, officials from the FDA's Vaccines and Related Biological Products Advisory Committee[35] discussed a new potential contaminant that allegedly had been found in bovine and human serum used for products such as children's injectable polio vaccines and Human Immune Globulin. The meeting participants listened as Dr. Dennis Kopecko, chief of one of the FDA laboratories, summarized the work of Kajander and his colleagues, who had suggested that such contamination may play a role in heart disease and kidney stones that are related to deposition of calcium in the human body.[36]

Kopecko explained that none of this contamination was likely to have occurred, because according to him, Dr. Kajander had misinterpreted the data.[37] The gene sequence found in tests by a team that Kopecko participated in resembled that of another type of bacterium, *Phyllobacterium*.[38] According to him, there was no credible molecular evidence to support the existence of nanobacteria.[39]

Furthermore, he believed that the other structures seen by his group and Kajander's were nonliving hydroxyapatite crystals, not nanobacteria.

Therefore, Kajander's identification of nanobacteria looked to Kopecko like a mistake.

THE CRITICS CRITICIZED

The idea that these might be "self-propagating microcrystalline apatite," as the Cisar team put it, was itself roundly slammed by other scientists. For example, Jorgen Christoffersen, who studies calcification at the University of Copenhagen in Denmark, said the self-propagating crystal claim was "scientific nonsense."[40] So the Cisar study was by no means universally accepted in the science community as being legitimate.

Despite this lack of agreement among scientists in the field, the possibility of such contamination was subsequently dismissed by the committee for the time being.[41]

In so doing, the committee depended heavily on the experiment and paper by John Cisar, Kopecko, and others,[42] which according to Kajander and Çiftçioğlu employed incomplete methods for characterizing the organisms. The Cisar team, they say, reached the right results by culturing the entities but did not use commercially available controlled culturing techniques and verifying methods to avoid contamination.[43] Kajander also says that Cisar had found only weak signs of DNA because nanobacteria have a special DNA strand that does not respond well to the type of detection methods used by Cisar.[44] The nucleic acid detection problem is especially relevant because it suggests again that nanobacteria have a unique nucleic acid structure, different from other known organisms.

Such issues had been discussed with the FDA earlier. Prior to the committee's regular session, a meeting had occurred between Kopecko's group and Kajander and Çiftçioğlu, in which possible reasons for the Cisar team findings were discussed. What was actually said at that meeting is disputed among attendees. Among the many contentious points, most focus on methods and interpretations used by each side.

Both teams claimed that the other's samples were contaminated.[45] The Cisar team found *Phyllobacterium* in its own tests and deduced from this that Kajander and Çiftçioğlu's tests were also contaminated with the bacterium. Wrong, say Çiftçioğlu and Kajander. Nanobacteria resemble *Phyllobacterium* in some ways, but they can be differentiated by structure, growth requirements, and biochemistry, which are accepted methods for telling organisms apart.

Some of this came back to nucleic acid. Kopecko said that there was none evident to support nanobacteria being special. Kajander countered that while the nucleic acid of nanobacteria had not been fully characterized, careful methods were required to isolate the type that set it apart from organisms such as *Phyllobacterium*. He said that the Cisar tests failed "because he did not use the best techniques and got all tests contaminated."[46]

Thus, everybody appeared to agree on one point: more nucleic acid testing was required.

Other scientists had produced studies claiming that nanobacteria couldn't be found, then concluded that they might not exist. In 2003 a group in France produced one such study. A telling element was that these researchers were unable to generate biofilm in their samples, although other researchers had reported being able to do so.[47] Nor did they mention the finding of nanobacteria by Mayo Clinic researchers in 2002. Moreover, according to Çiftçioğlu, they did not consult with her team on methodologies for the tests.[48]

Another claim made against Kajander and Çiftçioğlu was that they refused to share their nanobacteria samples and therefore were their own worst enemies by slowing independent research. The two scientists bristled at these accusations, pointing to more than a dozen labs that they said had already received samples and had published results. The underlying problem, they explained, was that some labs are not certified to deal with biohazards, and because nanobacteria pose an infection risk, it would have been irresponsible to hand out samples to every lab that requested them. As an example of the risks involved, they cite the transmission of the fatal SARS virus among researchers in several labs in Asia. Due to such risks, Çiftçioğlu said that it took her up to a year to get NASA to accept nanobacteria samples for testing.[49]

Still other critics claimed that Kajander and Çiftçioğlu's earlier incorporation of a company to sell tests for nanobacteria compromised their scientific objectivity.[50] If so, then many leading scientists in most every field of science had also been compromised because commercial exploitation of scientific discovery had by then grown commonplace and was often encouraged by universities instead of frowned upon. So the criticism appeared especially strange because such a practice was nothing out of the ordinary.

Then there were claims that Kajander and Çiftçioğlu had never shown clear photographs of nanobacteria, so it was hard to know what they were talking about. That claim was also false, because as early as 1998, clear photographs of nanobacteria had been published by the National Academy of Sciences as shown in figure 6.

Finally, some skeptics said that Kajander had never explained why nanobacteria varied so much in size from 50 nanometers to up to a micron.

But again, by 1998 he had published an explanation, with accompanying photographs. These demonstrated that the slow calcification of nanobacteria, plus their subsequent ability to form calcified colonies, led to the size variance.[51]

Just about every accusation, from contamination to greed and scientific error, was being thrown at the discoverers. Oddly though, few critics were stepping forward to validate the criticisms in experiments. Scientists who often had no lab experience with nanobacteria were shooting from the gallery without substantiating their positions. And some media were using those positions to discount high-level laboratory studies about nanobacteria. For Kajander and Çiftçioğlu, it was like fighting a persistent ghost.

What makes nanobacteria so special?

In the absence of complete nucleic acid identification, what made nanobacteria alive or special? According to Kajander's team, among the characteristics are differing reactions to antibiotics, disinfectants, and radiation (see fig. 7).

The researchers also pointed out why nanobacteria and the resulting calcium deposits can't come from nonliving crystalline processes:

- Nanobacteria calcify when calcium concentrations are low, whereas nonbiological crystals grow when calcium concentrations are high.

- The formation of a biofilm from cultured nanobacteria shows that they self-replicate as living cells do.

- Nanobacteria grow when exposed to certain light, whereas nonliving crystals do not.[52]

- Nanobacteria grow in the media used to produce cell cultures, but nonliving apatite crystals dissolve in the same media.[53]

- Doses of antibiotics or gamma radiation stop biofilm production by nanobacteria. This suggests that their biofilm-generating capacities have been neutralized. This strongly suggests that lifelike processes had to exist in the first place to be interrupted.

In view of such evidence, it seems odd that prior to discounting nanobacteria as a potential problem in vaccines, the FDA group did not suggest that experiments be conducted under independent monitoring.

Property	Human nanobacteria	Viral particles	Prion particles	Bacteria
Size [nm]	50-300	20-250	<250	>250
Self-replicating	Yes	No	No	Yes
Resistance to gamma irradiation [mrad]	~2.5	<2.5	>2.5	<0.1->6.0
Resist boiling	Yes	No	Yes	No
Resist disinfectants	Yes	Some	Yes	No
Resist antibiotics	Most all	Yes	Yes	Resistant to some
Cause inflammation	Yes	Yes	No	Yes
Cause host cell death	Yes	Yes	Specific	Some
Cause pathologic calcification	Yes	A few	No	A few
Form biofilms	Yes	No	No	Yes
Found in athero-sclerotic plaque	Yes	Some	No	A few

Figure 7: *How to tell* **Nanobacterium sanguineum**. *Here are a few defining characteristics of human nanobacteria that, according to their discoverers, make them special. This table shows how they are similar to, and different from, other types of pathogens.* [Table adapted from Katja Aho and E. Olavi Kajander, "Pitfalls in the Detection of Novel Nanoorganisms," Letters to the Editor, *Journal of Clinical Microbiology* 41, no. 7 (July 2003): 3460–61.]

The logic of "don't investigate" grew more questionable as other institutions published findings of nanobacteria in disease. Scientists at the University of Illinois found them in kidney and brain disease, as we'll discuss later. Mayo Clinic researchers reported that they identified nanobacteria-like structures in human arterial plaque,[54] confirming results produced earlier by Hungarian Academy of Sciences researcher László Puskás.[55] Then in 2004, Mayo researchers published more findings, demonstrating that nucleic acid formation observed with nanobacteria is generated by a process normally seen only in living organisms.[56]

The reluctance to investigate was also perplexing because no FDA-approved drug had been very successful at reversing calcification in various diseases. This was partly because no certain cause had been found.

Therefore, why would the FDA not want to encourage such investigations to see whether the earlier findings had merit?

WHAT IF THEY ARE RIGHT?

Such findings posed a serious challenge to the FDA advisory committee conclusions and raised a troubling question: what if Çiftçioğlu and Kajander were right about vaccine contamination?

On one hand, the agency could justifiably argue that its decision had conformed with regulations and that much evidence was so far circumstantial. However, on the other hand, was it possible that something slipped past the filtering and sterilization techniques used to protect vaccines against contamination? Although rare, it wouldn't be unprecedented. Some viruses eluded capture in blood serum for many years.[57]

Despite such worries, Kajander and Çiftçioğlu emphasized that this was not a reason to stop getting vaccinations. In their view, because nanobacteria are slow growing they are less immediately dangerous compared to the effects of diseases that vaccines prevent.

IT STARTED WITH THE KIDNEYS

In the related controversy over whether calcium deposits come from nanobacteria, some of the most intriguing evidence is found in the kidneys.

About one in ten persons develops kidney stones in a lifetime. When stones get stuck in the urinary tract or begin to move along it, they can instantly debilitate the strongest individual.

Kidney stone prevalence has risen for twenty years among Americans and Europeans, but no one knows why. The cause of most stones is also still unknown, although it has been linked to diet, lifestyle, and heredity.[58] Once someone has them, he or she is prone to getting them again. This is especially true with patients who have stones surgically removed or pulverized by shock wave therapy.[59]

Calcium deposits that make up most of these stones form a jagged series of outcroppings, known as "spicules," around a solid core. When they move down the urinary tract, these spurs scrape the nerves raw and also cause the stone to stick in the passageway. Calcification plays a part in most stone formation. A rarer stone, known as a "struvite," is caused by another well-known infection in the urinary tract.[60] However, this is not the case with most stones.

One explanation for how the most common stones form is that for unknown reasons, crystals of calcium stick to the insides of the kidneys.

Normally these are excreted in urine, but in some cases they are not. These calcium crystals congregate to form stones.[61]

THE IGLOO

Researchers have noticed for decades that as kidney stones form, the crystalline structures near their core have a hollow "igloo" shape to them.[62] Such a shape is normally seen when living organisms are present. This suggests infection.

In 1996, Neva Çiftçioğlu's brother Vefa Çiftçioğlu, a Turkish dentist who had been researching nanobacteria in periodontal disease, urged her to investigate the link between nanobacteria and kidney stones. He had developed stones, although there was no history of them in the family. He suspected that he had been infected.

When Neva Çiftçioğlu began examining dissected stones through an electron microscope, she found at the heart of them the same igloo-like structures that she'd seen growing years ago in a petri dish of cultured nanobacteria (see fig. 6). Most of the cores of these stones tested positive for nanobacteria.

In 1998 Çiftçioğlu and Kajander reported those findings in the *Proceedings of the National Academy of Sciences*[63] and theorized that nanobacteria were acting as "nidi" (centers) in kidney stone formation.

Just prior to that, University of Illinois researchers Drs. Thomas Hjelle and Marcia Miller-Hjelle had read about Kajander's work and contacted him to suggest collaborative investigation of polycystic kidney disease (PKD). This hereditary disease, affecting millions worldwide, results in cysts that cause the kidneys to swell and eventually stop working. When that happens, dialysis and transplants are the only treatments.[64]

As with heart disease, microbes had been suspected of triggering PKD, but no one was able to isolate them. The evidence pointing to an infection was even stronger than in heart disease because toxins from bacteria had often been identified in the fluid that came from such cysts.[65]

The Hjelles extracted fluid from the cysts and checked for nanobacterial antibodies and antigens. Nanobacterial antigens were found in 75 percent of the cases, and the nanobacteria themselves were cultured from many of the specimens.[66]

This work by University of Illinois and University of Edinburgh experts was crucial because it took the medical study of nanobacteria into some of the most respected medical institutions and made it hard for critics to claim that findings were restricted to just a few researchers. As the circle of investigators widened, the possibility of a fraudulent or mistaken claim was becoming less probable.

THE CASE OF RANDALL'S PLAQUES

Earlier in 1998 Çiftçioğlu, Kajander, and the Hjelles also met with University of Chicago Professor Fredric Coe, founder of a testing and disease management service for kidney stone patients. Coe, a leading kidney stone researcher and practitioner, was noted for his success in reducing kidney stone recurrence in patients.

According to Kajander and Çiftçioğlu, when they showed him photographs of the igloo-like structures, Coe went to his library and brought back a journal article published decades earlier by Dr. Alexander Randall, a pioneering kidney researcher known for identifying formations named "Randall's Plaques." The article described those same igloo-like structures in the plaques. Çiftçioğlu maintained that this special igloo was central to whether nanobacteria existed and were alive. She said that the detection and culturing of nanobacteria from the core of such structures refuted the argument that a nonliving crystalline process produced them.

Coe began to examine kidney stone cores as part of a multimillion-dollar NIH-funded study that had gone on for some years.[67] By 2003, as part of that work, his team produced evidence that the smallest pieces of plaque in kidneys were composed of calcium phosphate.[68] This was the same material that the Hjelles had found in the igloo-like structures. Was there a link? Coe didn't speculate, but it was clear from his research that some dominant theories about kidney stone formation were being rewritten.

Coe wasn't the only one to study such formations. Mayo Clinic researchers were also investigating nanobacteria in kidney stones, having identified them in their own independent analysis earlier.[69]

VERIFICATION FROM INDIA

In 2004 an independent team working at a university in India published in the journal *Urological Research* an experiment that replicated Çiftçioğlu's earlier work by finding nanobacteria in kidney stone patients and culturing the organisms from samples. The researchers also found indirect evidence of DNA. They concluded:

> We have enough evidence to suggest that these microparticles are living microorganisms . . . The presence of nanobacteria in kidney stones suggests that these bacteria may be involved in the etiology [cause] of such stones.[70]

Those findings made it increasingly hard for skeptics to deny the existence of a self-replicating nano-organism that had its own DNA structure and that triggered disease. However, the description in that paper of nanobacteria as "bacteria"—cited from an older study—perpetuated discussion over their genus.[71]

SOLVING A SERIOUS CASE OF MISTAKEN IDENTITY

In their kidney investigations, Kajander, Çiftçioğlu, and the Hjelles discovered a feature of nanobacteria that would solve another mystery for medical researchers but this time relating to heart disease.

Many bacteria and viruses have been identified in arterial plaque. One of those is *Chlamydia pneumoniae*, a bacterium tied to lung infections. For years a commonly applied commercial test has been used to find evidence of *Chlamydia*. However, there has been a problem with the test. Once scientists found the indicator, they often could not culture the germ from the plaque. This was important because *Chlamydia* had been implicated as a potential contributor to heart disease, yet often its presence could not be confirmed. Many studies note this contradiction.

While looking for nanobacteria in kidney stones, the University of Illinois team came up with a remarkable finding: nanobacteria give off a "false positive" for *Chlamydia* when the commercial test is used.[72] The same cross-reactivity was found for a bacterium known as *Bartonella*, which has also been detected in heart disease. Thus, for years scientists may have been getting false positives generated by nanobacteria, when they thought that they were detecting *Chlamydia* or *Bartonella*. This explains why sometimes they couldn't culture *Chlamydia* and *Bartonella*. In those cases, they just weren't there.

This does not mean that *Chlamydia* and *Bartonella* aren't players in kidney or heart disease. Instead, it suggests that nanobacteria precede or accompany them and may be present when the other pathogens aren't.

CORRECTING ERRONEOUS TECHNIQUES

Ironically, critics used the false positive to argue that something else was being mistaken for nanobacteria, when research suggested it was the other way around. Kajander explained that the false positive gave the first logical explanation for why organisms such as *Chlamydia* bacteria couldn't be cultured when tests suggested they were present. They simply were not there. Instead, researchers may have been finding nanobacteria and misidentifying them due to the false positive. This again demonstrated why nanobacteria were masters of disguise and had confounded attempts to pin them down.

Exasperated by the defective methods being used to find nanobacteria, Kajander, with his colleague and wife, Katja Aho, as lead author, published a paper on how to avoid the procedural pitfalls so that researchers could accurately describe the particles.[73] See figure 7 for properties of human nanobacteria compared to other pathogens, and see figure 8 for a list of discoveries about the special characteristics.

The Remarkable Discoveries

Human nanobacteria
- Are found in human blood
- Replicate much more slowly than most viruses or bacteria
- Require special methods to observe and culture them
- Uniquely form a hard calcium phosphate shell in blood-like conditions
- Resist radiation and heat that kill most bacteria and viruses
- Trigger the same type of swelling and clotting found in heart disease and injuries
- Cause kidney stones in lab animals injected with them
- Contaminate vaccines and slip through conventional filters
- Lead researchers to mislabel them by emitting a "false positive" for other infections
- Have been found in arterial plaque, heart valves, ovarian cancer, dental stones, and kidney stones
- Have been found in every heart disease patient who participated in a clinical trial
- Are a reliable indicator of coronary artery calcification
- Are treatable with a novel combination of well-known chemicals and drugs

---

Figure 8: *The remarkable discoveries. This plain-language list shows what had to be found out before researchers could understand what nanobacteria are and do. Some of those properties are described earlier in this chapter, while others are covered in later chapters. Taken together, they show why so much time was required to uncover the disease-related properties of this pathogen, especially with so few resources available for early investigations.*

As more research was being published about nanobacteria, some scientists also tried to get away from the name that had been given to the pathogen so that their peers would not dismiss the research based on a misunderstanding of one word. Substitutes such as "self-replicating nanoparticles" and "nanobes" began to be used more frequently. Sometimes the term "nanobacteria" was nowhere to be found in research that described them. And because so many preconceptions had been formed about nanobacteria in the science funding community, researchers investigating the particles had to call them something else to be considered for financial support. All of these gymnastics came about because some critics opposed the idea that nanobacteria might be alive and refused to support work that aimed to determine whether they were or not.

WHAT TRULY MATTERS TO PATIENTS

Does it matter if nanobacteria are alive or not in the accepted sense? To thousands of researchers it matters very much because this is the stuff of Nobel Prizes—defining the limits of life or finding new organisms with deep implications for the ecology and microbiology.

Imagine, for example, if nanobacteria were shown to be ubiquitous in the environment. Our ideas of how ecosystems function might have to be rethought. We might have to consider that a whole universe of organisms underpins the one that we are used to dealing with. For the human body, concepts of what lives in the blood and how the body deals with infectious organisms might have to be revised.

However, one pressing issue overshadows those debates. Regardless of what nanobacteria are, something doesn't have to be "alive" in the regular sense to cause trouble in the body. For example, arguments continue over whether viruses are "alive." Some researchers argue that these cannot replicate on their own; therefore, they aren't living organisms.[74] Still, they contain RNA and DNA, and they cause no end of harm. Likewise, tiny protein particles known as "prions," some of which are thought to cause mad cow disease (BSE), are not considered to be alive, yet they too cause much trouble and can kill.

The arguments over whether nanobacteria live may testify to an ingenious survival strategy. As we'll see, they work as cagey catalysts that allow other diseases to take hold. While researchers argue over what category the marauders fall into, nanobacteria seem to knock down the gates of immunity in countless human victims.

Whether alive or dead, organisms or not, it's not so much what they *are* as what they *do*. It is their effects, not their classification, that stump doctors and terrify patients. For those doctors and patients, as we'll see in the next chapters, here is what truly matters:

- ▣ Nanobacteria don't care what we call them; they still seem to harm us in great numbers.

- ▣ Human nanobacteria are found in the calcified deposits that permeate arterial plaque, kidney stones, and other disease sites. Patients with these diseases often test positive for the pathogen.

- ▣ Calcium deposits associated with nanobacteria are found in the body and are toxic. They do not have to be alive to kill a human. The most important step is to get rid of them.

Five

Seeds of Destruction

By 2002 scientists from high profile research institutes were hot on the trail of human nanobacteria and had published the makings of an apparently great discovery:

> [We found] evidence of nanometer-scale structures in calcified human cardiovascular tissue. These structures are similar to nanobacteria described and isolated from human kidney stones and geological specimens. These observations fulfill one criterion for Koch's postulate [sic] to suggest that a calcifying "nanobe" could participate in calcification of vascular tissue.[1]

Thus, investigators from the Mayo Clinic and University of Texas confirmed what Hungarian researcher László Puskás had found earlier. Nanobacteria are in heart disease. That finding received more support when a related group at Mayo concluded in 2004 that newer data "suggest that viable nano-sized organisms are present within calcified human arterial tissue."[2]

Around the same time, another quiet bombshell came from different researchers based in Charleston, West Virginia, who positively identified nanobacteria in a calcified heart valve of an end-stage diabetes patient.[3]

Despite that, there was nothing new about finding infections in heart disease and cancers. As we'll see, many infections have already been identified, but it doesn't mean that they cause the illness.

Mindful of that history, the Mayo researchers added cautiously: "A cause and effect relationship between the presence of these organisms and development of arterial calcification remains to be determined."[4]

However, unknown to them, other researchers were about to show an association between nanobacteria and heart disease.

SMOKING GUNS OR CIRCUMSTANTIAL EVIDENCE?

In April 2004, researchers at the Cardiovascular Research Institute, Washington Hospital Center in Washington, D.C., reported that patients with extensive calcification in their coronary arteries also had significant amounts of nanobacteria. Because the level of arterial calcification is a good predictor of heart disease, this suggested that a nanobacteria test was also a good predictor.[5]

Did it mean that nanobacteria cause coronary artery calcification? Not necessarily. They could just be there by coincidence and grow as the calcification increases.

Still, evidence pointed to it being more than coincidence. First was the growth rate of nanobacteria in relation to the calcification rate. Compared to other viruses and bacteria found in heart disease, the replication rate of nanobacteria is very slow—as is the calcification rate in arteries. This, say some researchers, may explain why calcification accumulates unnoticeably in its early stages and why the tortoise-like pace has never matched the growth rate of other infections that scientists isolated in heart disease.[6]

The doubling of calcium deposits every few years may also explain why so many patients who have no apparent signs of heart disease get sick or die suddenly. In a young adult the doubling of a tiny growth might go unnoticed for decades. But then in its later stages, such a doubling may cause significant blockage.

But the accumulation alone wouldn't explain such drastic changes in so many unsuspecting victims over a few weeks or days. The added element is swelling triggered by those same calcium phosphate crystals. When passages are partially blocked, swelling and clots can be, and often are, fatal. For example, when calcium phosphate crystals are released due to a rupture of plaque, an artery might go from being only slightly blocked by plaque to completely plugged by rapid inflammation and clotting.

This combined onslaught might also explain why doctors often find that arterial blockage has occurred in an area that was not previously detected as a potential trouble spot.

Then we come back to a question posed earlier: *Why do we calcify when our blood calcium level is normal?*

Nanobacteria seem to be the only known pathogens to grow a calcified shell when calcium is not plentiful and acidity is neutral.[7] Kajander and his colleagues found that they suck calcium from their surroundings, then combine it with other chemicals and compounds, such as cholesterol or lipids, to secrete biofilm.[8] Çiftçioğlu found that this solidifies into apatite, a calcium compound armor.

The capacity to generate such a shell under regular blood-like conditions seems unique to nanobacteria. The ability to do that when low and moderate concentrations of calcium are present may explain why we calcify when our calcium blood levels are balanced.

Is it possible that another organism could be responsible for this? It's doubtful, say researchers. Some conventional bacteria can generate calcium carbonate,[9] another form of calcification, but none are known to manufacture calcium phosphate under such conditions.[10]

Once nanobacteria are encased in their shell, they go semidormant. On casual examination they look like microscopic snowballs (see fig. 6). The shell is hard to strip off. It resists high heat, radiation, and drugs. Someone can examine it under an electron microscope yet without training not see the nanobacteria that are in it. This has led some to dismiss the shell as a calcium "artifact."

However, the findings by the Mayo Clinic and Washington Hospital Center of nanobacteria in heart disease suggest that this is no artifact. Instead, a plausible mechanism has been found for calcium deposits in atherosclerosis and the swelling that accompanies them.

WHEN SOMETHING IS A CAUSE OF DISEASE

What other evidence is there that nanobacteria cause disease? The rules observed by every medical scientist for proving the link between an organism and disease are known as "Koch's Postulates," developed by physician and bacteriologist Robert Koch around the turn of the twentieth century:

- The microorganism must be detectable in the infected host at every stage of the disease.

- The microorganism must be isolated from the diseased host and grown in pure culture.

- When susceptible, healthy animals are infected with pathogens from the pure culture, the specific symptoms of the disease must occur.

◙ The microorganism must be reisolated from the diseased animal and correspond to the original microorganism in pure culture.

Have these conditions been met for nanobacteria? Not yet in heart disease, but apparently for the kidneys. In 2000 and 2001, Spanish scientist Enrique Garcia-Cuerpo and a team of researchers published papers in the Spanish *Journal of Urology* outlining how they had met each condition by injecting nanobacteria into healthy laboratory animals, then tracing them through the metabolism, finding them in excreted urine, detecting them in kidney damage, and culturing the extracted nanobacteria from resulting kidney stone samples.[11] Furthermore, Kajander and his team discovered similar evidence in human subjects.[12]

Do nanobacteria trigger heart disease?

At the time of writing, no definitive study had been published showing laboratory evidence of the whole sequence by which nanobacteria may trigger the atherosclerotic process. So what is the point in talking about nanobacteria in heart disease? Isn't this just premature speculation?

Far from it, say researchers. A careful examination of published studies shows a remarkable similarity between heart disease and the processes that nanobacteria and their calcium crystals generate:

◙ Nanobacteria produce the same type of calcium deposits that are found in the hard and soft plaque deposits of atherosclerosis. Nanobacteria and calcium deposits have also been found together in atherosclerotic plaque.

◙ These deposits are well known to be toxic, generating the same type of inflammation found in atherosclerosis and many other diseases.

◙ Nanobacteria replicate at a turtle's pace compared to other microorganisms. This rate is more comparable to the formation rate of atherosclerotic plaque than to the replication rate of other infections found in heart disease.

◙ Virtually every atherosclerosis patient who has undergone tests for nanobacteria has been shown to have them. By contrast, the infection rate in generally healthy populations has been found to be much lower. Moreover, a statistical correlation has been established between the level of coronary artery calcification and nanobacterial infection in patients.

▣   As we'll see later, a formula has been devised that eradicates
       nanobacteria by targeting the same calcium deposits that are
       found in heart disease. We'll also see that when heart patients are
       treated for nanobacteria, they show measurable improvement as
       nanobacteria and accompanying calcium deposits are removed.

A theoretical framework has been developed for how nanobacteria
might work in heart disease.[13] This is included later as an appendix. See
"How Nanobacteria May Trigger the Atherosclerotic Process."

WHAT ABOUT CANCER?

Evidence that nanobacteria-grown calcium crystals may trigger cancer is
less developed, but there are undeniable links.

As described in chapter 1, calcification is a dependable marker and early
warning sign of many cancers. Some calcified deposits in the breasts are
associated with malignancy.[14] One property of such deposits is to make
cells replicate rapidly.[15]

The crystals have another habit: they stimulate absorption of DNA
by cells from their surroundings. This may lead to inflammation and cell
death.[16] Inflammation is a concern because it is often found at cancer
sites. Nanobacteria that generate such inflammation-inducing calcification have been identified in tumors of ovarian cancer patients.[17]

WHERE DO NANOBACTERIA COME FROM?

What are the sources of nanobacteria, and can we stop them before they
contaminate us? The list of possible origins is long and underinvestigated.
Everything from Martian meteorites to underground or underwater repositories has been suggested. Because nanobacteria are in livestock, this
suggests that they come from an environmental source.[18] Many people eat
red meat, and because calcium-encased nanobacteria may not be eradicated
by cooking, they might enter us that way. Urine from infected animals and
humans has high nanobacteria levels and may contaminate drinking water
sources. One study suggests that similar particles are in some water supplies.[19] Due to their small size and resilience, they may evade conventional
purification. They slip through nanofilters, for example.

Studies have not yet been published on the presence of nanobacteria in
plants, so it is not certain if we are infected when we eat these.

Nanobacteria may be distributed throughout our environment, but
whether we develop disease from that depends on how many contaminated
sources we are exposed to and our genetic abilities to fight infection.

One area where it may be possible to stop the contamination is with fetal bovine serum, the same medium that Kajander used to find nano-bacteria in the 1980s:

> How are humans exposed to nanobacteria? Cows seem to be hosts to nanobacteria and biopharmaceutical products from cell culture (fetal bovine serum used as a supplement) are occasionally contaminated with nanobacteria. Such a contamination has been recently reported in viral vaccines. About 15% of human serum samples from healthy blood donors contain anti-nanobacteria antibodies and nanobacteria can be occasionally found and cultured from serum . . . As the first phase we screened presence of nanobacteria markers in 7 commercial gamma globulin products. We found that nanobacteria antigen was culturable in 2 out of 7 preparations studied.[20]

Is such contamination a problem?[21] Does it seem to be life-threatening? Is it possible to stop nanobacteria by filtering fetal bovine serum? Is there some link with beef-related diseases? These are good questions. As more researchers begin to find nanoscale organisms, and with discovery of why mammalian cells die in fetal bovine serum, it seems prudent to start looking for other possible sources of entry into the human body.

Right now the more immediate issue is, How do we get rid of the bad calcification that's already in us and that poses a clear threat?

Part II
Containing an Explosion

Six
When to Declare "I'm Safe"

M ost calcific diseases are treatable but incurable. We can beat them back but in the end, they get to us. If we could shift that paradigm in our favor, then medicine and our lives might be transformed.

To bring about such a transition we must carefully consider what it means to be "cured." In plain terms, being cured means getting rid of an illness so that it doesn't come back, then also being restored to good health. This may seem obvious, but actually there are many definitions of a cure, from finding no trace of an infection over a few weeks to being free of cancer for years.[1]

We can be cured of an illness but still be stuck with the effects. This is the case with leprosy, for example, where patients may be cured but still suffer internal or external scars. Such lingering damage must also be considered with "cures" for other illnesses.

Nowhere is this more apparent than with the terminal illness of heart disease.

THE HOLY GRAIL

Heart disease is now on the rampage. Its presence in ancient mummies shows that it has stalked us for millennia, but it has erupted as a scourge only in the last century. Its tentacles touch more than half a billion of us. It is typically fatal regardless of how well or early it is treated.

To beat one of the most prevalent types—atherosclerosis—doctors will have to fix what comes with it.[2] An early indicator is inflammation that narrows blood vessels. The next is soft and hard plaque: a gooey substance comprised of fats, fiber, and calcified deposits that we know as "hardening of the arteries." Finally there is clotting; a normally healthy process that harms us when it occurs in arteries.

Nor does a cause or cure necessarily start with the heart. First, the tiny capillaries that make up most of our circulatory system start to plug. By the time we sense a problem, these have been sick for a while.

Therefore, to conquer the illness, doctors have to confront it at the invisible starting gate. That is why stopping it when patients are in their twenties and thirties is so vital, because this is when the trouble starts.

There are so many battles: try to prevent it when patients are young, treat it effectively when they are old, and just plain get rid of it. Is there a link that might help us to do these together?

A QUESTIONABLE BASIS FOR TREATMENT

Many theories are offered for how to cure hardening of the arteries, but until now no one has given proof in an independently verified clinical trial. The quest has been haunted by a triple curse. First, no published methods have reversed the fatal combination of inflammation, clotting, and buildup in blood vessels. Drugs and diets may slow it, but none sustainably reverses it. Next, no one has shown why calcium ends up in the wrong places, causing arteries to stiffen and organs to malfunction. Finally, signs of infection keep popping up, but no contagious "smoking gun" has been found: possible culprits, yes; convicted criminals, no.

This may explain why *half of fatal heart attacks occur with no apparent prior symptoms.*[3] The other half are anticipated and often treated but not prevented. Doctors and drug companies continue to care for the symptoms instead of the cause of the most prevalent terminal disease in existence.[4]

COSTS OF TREATING JUST SYMPTOMS

Because medical science didn't find a culprit, most resources have been spent on controlling its worst effects. Experts are trained to control the pain and crippling conditions. Surgeons physically cut out or patch the most dangerous carnage. Pharmacists, researchers, and psychologists help victims to cope with the fallout. Governments and foundations spend great sums researching how to reduce the impacts of the disease. A gigantic drug and dietary supplement infrastructure surrounds this. Anticholesterol drugs saturate patients' bloodstreams, while advertisements for them permeate the brain. Blood thinners, antistroke and high blood pressure medication, and fat-free diets are used to alleviate symptoms. Ultimately, it's an expensive, hard-fought but losing battle. Most of the time, this defensive army only manages to delay the inevitable.

Just as worrisome, the costs of this war are gutting family, corporate, and government finances, causing economic havoc that is more profound than most other threats that politicians and economists have us worry about.

And there is another cost. Much of the progress in treating symptoms is based on patients taking drugs for the rest of their lives. In many cases, the side effects of these lifelong treatments are serious and can lead to complications. Drugs help patients to cope, but at what price to them, their families, and the healthcare infrastructure?

Treating symptoms helps to keep us going, but the U.S. Surgeon General describes why the supporting framework—which outstrips the American military in size—is a financial albatross around the necks of patients, businesses, and governments:

> Heart disease not only attacks our hearts; it places a burden on our healthcare system. It accounts for 29 percent of all hospitalizations, more than a third of all nursing home care, and 23 percent of hospice care. It also affects our chances of longevity. If we could eliminate heart disease, the life expectancy of the average American would increase by five years![5]

SLOWING IT DOESN'T REVERSE IT

Perhaps due to this massive investment of money and reputations in treating symptoms, claims about cures for heart disease are often met with the same skepticism by doctors as a claim that snake oil cures gout.

Many conventional and alternative "cures" are based on diets, vitamins, or chemical removal of toxins from the body. There is evidence that some of these delay or reduce the symptoms. The term "reverse heart disease" is also used, but this is often a misstatement. Partial reversal might occur with the symptoms but not with the cause—and usually not with the ultimate results.

There is also a difference between reversal and *slowing the rate of progression*. Drugs, diets, and surgery may retard the pace. Surgeons cut out obstructions, but these can recur. Specially treated stents prevent reblockage of artery repairs, but these are only partially effective.[6] Drugs known as "statins" have been successful at combating blockage, but these seem to slow rather than reverse the process.[7]

SHOOTING AT FOOTPRINTS

The depth of desperation over "reversing" heart disease was typified by the attention lavished on an announcement in 2003 of a "polypill" that promised to cram many symptom-reducing drugs into one daily pill.[8] Despite the pill not existing and not being tried, manufactured, approved, or applied to the proposed target population, researchers claimed it would cut heart attacks by about 80 percent. While medical associations and cardiologists pointed out "massive caveats" to the untried concept of saturating the whole human population over fifty-five years of age with such a combination, the idea still garnered intense publicity as a potential solution—a virtually done deal.[9]

Shortly after that, hopes were raised again by a study of a small group of patients who were injected with a synthesized variant of cholesterol known as "HDL" that was suspected to prevent heart disease. The study claimed that scientists had achieved significant regression of dangerous plaque in the arteries.[10] This finding was based primarily on visual observations of arteries in each patient. Regardless of that, news reports interpreted this to mean that for the first time, heart disease had been *measurably reversed*.[11] However, the dependability and sustainability of these apparent reductions remained to be seen. For example, there did not seem to be evidence that the hard calcium deposits in arteries had been affected. Therefore, it was a stretch to say that heart disease, including all of its attendant symptoms, had been reversed.

Other research shows that many of us may be genetically disposed to heart disease and that genetic therapies may help to prevent it.[12] The question remains, disposed to *what*? Exactly what do our genes lack in these cases? Researchers don't know if turning on one gene might leave us open to something else. The analogy is to correct a line of code in a software program, only to find that the correction makes the program malfunction somewhere else.

All of these approaches have been admirable for their preventative strategies. Some may already be helping to reduce or postpone death from heart disease. They are certainly not to be discounted.

Nonetheless, by attempting to stop the problem without knowing the cause, every heart disease treatment has been shooting at the footprints of an invisible enemy.

DIET, EXERCISE, AND ALTERNATIVE THERAPIES

Many doctors tell their patients that losing weight, exercising, and eating the right foods cuts the chances for heart attacks. Evidence shows that weight loss and exercise improve your odds. Exactly what are the "right" foods for a healthy heart remains debatable. Among the prominent and controversial dietary or supplement methods claimed to prevent or fix heart disease have been Dr. Atkins' New Diet Revolution,[13] the South Beach Diet,[14] Dr. Dean Ornish's Program for Reversing Heart Disease,[15] Dr. Rath's Ten Step Program for Cardiovascular Health,[16] and the Linus Pauling unified theory of heart disease.[17]

Ironically, while some such approaches were being harshly criticized for straying too far from a "balanced" diet, U.S. government authorities were busy revising the traditional "food pyramid" that was recommended for years in America as the unassailable basis for such a balance. Why? Because that pyramid has also been lambasted for putting too much emphasis on some foods.[18]

Other methods such as stress management and meditation are said to work against heart disease and are often recommended in concert with diet and exercise. Intravenous chelation therapy, which involves extracting toxic metals from the blood, has also been used and is under intensive investigation, as we'll see later.[19]

Each has its own validity. Some such therapies are in opposition to each other. Still, many users swear by their results. Just because they may not be clinically verified yet doesn't mean they don't work. As we'll see in later chapters, some of them may bolster the body's own defenses.[20]

Yet so far, no diet, drug, or therapy has shown clinical trial evidence of reversing every measurable indicator of heart disease, including inflammation, clotting, and soft and hard plaques that contain calcium deposits.

THE INFECTIOUS CULPRITS?

The idea that most forms of cancer, heart disease, kidney stones, cataracts, and arthritis are *not* infection related has underpinned Western treatments since the mid-twentieth century. Most physicians, clinics, emergency rooms, hospitals, pharmacies, drug companies, and insurance plans work under that assumption. A good chunk of the globalized economy—in the form of a multitrillion-dollar medical industry—is predicated on the concept that infection is not responsible for most of the chronic diseases that kill us.

However, historically, just a handful of remarkable innovations relating to infection has defeated many diseases and dramatically improved human longevity. One was the discovery of a link between bacteria and infection.[21] This led to what is still one of the best disease prevention methods: washing our hands. Another was the vaccine, which controlled or eradicated infections (such as smallpox, diphtheria, and tuberculosis) that made humanity miserable for millennia.

A mixed bag of viruses, bacteria, and other lifelike substances occupy our arteries at one time or another. The walls of blood vessels seem to turn into garbage dumps where pathogens thrive. Bugs such as those that cause pneumonia have been fingered as heart disease culprits.[22] Studies have also found that patients who are infected with the herpes simplex virus, which causes cold sores, face a greater likelihood of heart attacks.[23] Various suspects in heart disease—and sometimes in cancer—are shown in figure 9, along with a few of the sicknesses that they are normally associated with.[24]

Throughout the centuries medical experts have theorized that heart disease is an infection, but the idea did not take hold in Western medical thinking until just a few years ago.[25] Why? Because no one had found a "smoking gun." Some books identify viruses and bacteria as causing coronary artery disease.[26] However, clinical trial evidence does not support this. Getting rid of the infections does not seem to reverse the illness.

CHECK YOUR TEETH

Gum disease is also mentioned frequently in figure 9. The links between oral and cardiac health are the subject of intense scrutiny by dentists and cardiologists. Studies have drawn a close correlation between periodontal disease and heart disease in some patients.[27] Therefore some dentists have started to pay attention to the general health of patients rather than just teeth, while some cardiologists look at teeth instead of just the heart.

That connection wasn't discovered suddenly. It emerged over years as physicians and dentists began to observe that heart patients had a history of gum disease. Knowledge about the link started to solidify only recently.

Such timelines show that Western medicine's understanding of the links between heart disease and other conditions has not been well developed; hence, the role of infection in heart disease may have been downplayed.

Some Pathogens Suspected in Heart Disease	
Bacteroides oralis	Bacteria in gum disease
Borrelia burgdorferi	Bacterial cause of Lyme disease
Chlamydia pneumoniae	Bacteria associated with pneumonia
Coxsackievirus	Virus associated with inflammation of the heart
Cytomegalovirus	Virus that can harm individuals who have low resistance
Epstein-Barr virus	Virus associated with infectious mononucleosis and cancer
Eubacterium alactolyticum	Bacteria in gum disease
Helicobacter pylori	Bacteria associated with gastric ulcer
Hepatitis A virus	Virus associated with liver infection
Herpes simplex virus type 2	Virus associated with primary genital infection and encephalitis
Mycoplasma fermentans and *Mycoplasma oralis*	Agent associated with gum disease
Mycoplasma genitalium	Agent associated with urogenital infection
Mycoplasma pneumoniae	Agent associated with pneumonia
Peptostreptococcus anaerobius	Bacteria in gum disease
Porphyromonas gingivalis	Bacteria in gum disease
Streptococcus sanguis and *Streptococcus oralis*	Bacteria in gum disease
Treponema pallidum	Bacterial cause of syphilis
Trypanozoma cruzi	Cause of Chagas' disease

Figure 9: *Some pathogens suspected in heart disease. Note that those such as strains of* Chlamydia *and the herpes virus are also implicated in cancer.*

THE USUAL SUSPECTS

Nonetheless, many pathogenic suspects have been found at the coronary crime scene and taken into custody. Some had charges against them dismissed for lack of evidence, despite their suspicious behavior. They have yet to be convicted for violence to the heart.

Clinical trial results for treatments of bacterial and viral infections in heart disease have been disappointing.[28] Despite that, the American Heart Association notes why researchers may be on to something:

> No one knows for sure what causes the low-grade inflammation that seems to put otherwise healthy people at risk. However, the new findings are consistent with the hypothesis that an infection—possibly one caused by a bacteria or a virus—might contribute to or even cause atherosclerosis ... Thus, it may be that antimicrobial or antiviral therapies will someday join other therapies used to prevent heart attacks.[29]

Furthermore, the association says that a disturbing precedent should make us pay more attention:

> This idea clearly needs to be tested in clinical trials. However, the notion that chronic infection can lead to unsuspected disease isn't foreign to most doctors. For example, bacterial infection with *Helicobacter pylori* is now known to be the major cause of stomach ulcers.[30]

RESISTING THE *IDEA* OF INFECTION

Evidence that heart disease could be triggered by a treatable infection seems like nonsense to some doctors. Why would they still be operating on millions of heart patients or prescribing drugs to relieve their suffering if someone had found a treatable infection that triggers the disease?

Yet in 1990, if that same question had been asked about stomach ulcers, similar responses could have been heard: Of course, stomach ulcers aren't triggered by an infection! Why would surgeons still be operating on tens of thousands of patients to fix ulcers if someone had found such a germ?

Ironically, by then researchers *had* found such a germ. And they knew the cure—a course of antibiotics. These had been discovered in the mid-1980s and the results published in medical journals. However, various medical agencies refused to acknowledge the proof for years.[31] Not until the mid-1990s did they adopt the treatment.[32]

If we get an ulcer, our physician may prescribe a drug to control bacteria that are causing the problem in our stomach. The bacterium, *Helicobacter pylori*, grows in us for years without causing much trouble, but then as we age it eats away at the walls of our digestive tract. If left for too long, it makes us bleed internally from an ulcer.

For years surgeons attacked this by cutting the nerve that goes from the brain to the abdomen and slicing open the small intestine to get at the ulcer. It was major surgery with a painful, slow recovery.

Then in 1982 two Australian researchers discovered that *Helicobacter pylori* was usually present in the stomach when an ulcer occurred. This is now commonly treated with antibiotics. Expensive and risky surgery is virtually never used anymore.[33]

But despite compelling scientific evidence, *it took from the mid-1980s until the mid-1990s for the approach to gain widespread acceptance*. In that interval, according to the Centers for Disease Control and Prevention in the United States, vast numbers of patients were prescribed ineffective drugs or underwent painful and unnecessary surgery.[34]

The stomach ulcer story is not an isolated example in medical history. Many treatments used today for a range of diseases took years to emerge from obscurity, while others were forgotten for centuries and then had to be rediscovered. Disinfection, which is credited as one of the greatest advances in improving human longevity, was practiced in an elementary form thousands of years ago by Egyptian and Greek physicians, then tragically lost to the Dark Ages until it was rediscovered in the nineteenth century.[35] After that, antibiotics that generated the next longevity revolution were ignored when first announced, then required years of research to be produced in bulk.[36]

These cases are well known to physicians and government authorities, but the question is, what has been learned?

Now, researchers have unearthed evidence of nanobacterial infection, with deep implications for patients who have heart and other diseases.[37] Has this too been overlooked, and if so, why? By downplaying the significance of these infectious signs, might critics of these discoveries have repeated history on a greater scale?

ARE GERMS THE CAUSE OR JUST OPPORTUNISTS?

Part of the reason for such stubbornness is that while many infections have been found in heart disease and cancer, it is still not clear as to *when* they take hold in the decades-long process and whether one of them is a primary trigger or an ongoing cause. For example, some studies show no correlation between infection and the onset of heart disease.[38] This suggests that instead of being at the root, many infections take hold later.

Other studies show that as multiple infections put more stress on the body, heart disease gets worse.[39] This is referred to as "total pathogen load." Once the body is weakened by such infections, it is open to diseases that gain a hold after earlier invasions have occurred. Therefore, while they may not be the triggers, infections that gang up on our heart still warrant serious attention. Doctors don't just write off such bugs because they aren't detected from the start. For example, some evaluations show that heart patients have a lower short-term recurrence of problems when treated with antibiotics.[40] This supports the idea that if infection can be fought off, then we might be able to beat heart disease.

Still, there is a problem. Doctors haven't *cured* heart disease by using antibiotics; they only temporarily alleviate a few symptoms. Why don't antibiotics that normally kill these organisms reverse heart disease? Are such infections secondary to an underlying problem? Did the attackers sneak in when the body's defenses were already weakened? Or were they there from the beginning?

Another paradox is that most such pathogens grow and replicate at a fast rate that can be monitored, so how could they drive a slow process such as atherosclerosis? Is it the same as with ulcers, where a bacterium triggers ulceration over time? Might we be continually reinfected so that the process degrades our resistance?

A mysterious underlying infection seems to be causing blood vessel irritation that comes and goes throughout our lives as the body's defenses, or medical treatments, struggle in vain to kill it.

GENETICS AND ENVIRONMENT

Heredity and environment also determine whether we can fight off such infection. Some of us may have natural immunity. Also, many environments are more "heart disease friendly" than others.

These factors are especially important because many persons who live a healthy lifestyle still get heart disease and die from it. Predisposition at a young age is the subject of intense genetic research. Scientists believe that they have found genes that make us more—or less—susceptible.[41]

Still, such susceptibility may not be the cause. It is only a sign that some of us are programmed to be more open, or react more or less severely, to that cause.

The genetic approach is not to be underestimated. Now that the human genome has been largely decoded, we can hope for remarkable discoveries about our susceptibility to many diseases.

The environments where we live and work also contribute to sparking or suppressing illness. Many studies show that some diseases are concentrated in geographic clusters. Kidney stones, some cancers, and other ailments are found in such clusters, but it is not always understood why.

To fully exploit the benefits of environmentally and genetically related therapies, doctors still have to know the triggers for these illnesses.

CAN A LINK BE MADE?

We've seen that heart disease doesn't show up in just one way. It involves thousands of chemical and biological interactions. These make a cure, an effective treatment, and prevention hard to achieve.

We've also seen that nanobacteria and resulting calcium crystals trigger many of the same symptoms that are present in heart disease. And they trigger the same type of inflammation that is found in many cancers. This opens a new range of possibilities, but only if their presence in disease can be measured.

The question is, can doctors test for them reliably in the human body and draw a meaningful link?

Seven

How Do I Know If I Have Them?

I t is hard to believe that with so much diagnostic medicine in our lives, and more of us having calcification than just about any other chronic condition, there has been no sure way for detecting calcium phosphate buildups with a blood test.[1] But until now, that has been the case.

Doctors do other tests for "ionized calcium," "calcium serum," and phosphorus, but these are usually to find elevated or low levels. This doesn't tell much about calcification because, as we've seen, it often happens when calcium blood levels are normal.

Here's the good news: this problem has been partially overcome. A quick blood test may now show who has coronary artery calcification and who is at serious risk of heart disease. Diagnostics that link nanobacteria with calcium phosphate deposits were verified in 2004 when researchers at Washington Hospital Center in Washington, D.C., found that the test is an accurate predictor of coronary calcification in patients.[2]

HOW DO THE TESTS WORK?

The body produces antibodies against nanobacteria just as it does with other types of disease. These antibodies can be used in tests to determine the presence of nanobacteria in blood and urine. A blood test was developed by Olavi Kajander and Neva Çiftçioğlu. The test supplies are sent to the patient's physician, who then draws the patient's blood and sends the sample to an assigned testing lab. Nanobacterial antigens show up on a scale of one to several thousand. A urine quick test has also been developed.[3]

Lab testing of randomly selected blood from residents in Finland has shown that a significant percentage of samples test positive for nanobacteria.[4] In separate analyses, every coronary heart disease patient who took the tests has also shown positive results for nanobacteria.[5]

The difficulty with depending only on these tests is that many of the dangerous nanobacteria in the body are dormant and surrounded by calcium, so they are undetectable. To further characterize such calcified deposits, other methods have to be used.

CALCIUM SCORING

One graphic representation of calcification in coronary artery disease comes from an ultrafast (or multislice) CT scan with calcification scoring. CT scan (or CAT scan) is the abbreviation for computerized axial tomography. The method uses x-rays to scan the body from different angles. Technicians take the information from those multiple x-rays and program a computer to generate pictures of thin slices of the body. The advantage of a CT scan over a regular x-ray is that, using the same level of radiation, it can show some soft tissue and other features that x-rays miss.[6]

Calcification is visible on a CT scan because it absorbs x-rays just like bones do. That area of the film remains underdeveloped. So, if you've got calcium deposits in your heart or other organs, these will usually show up.

In the late 1970s, CT scanning was so revolutionary that its inventors were awarded the Nobel Prize.[7] Today it is done routinely, and the accuracy is greatly improved. Without this improvement, it would be hard to see calcification in parts of the body.

Some small risks are associated with these low-dose ultrafast CT scans. As with every method that uses x-rays, too much exposure can generate cell mutations that lead to cancer because radiation is cumulative over your lifetime. However, it is generally accepted that the benefits of an occasional CT scan usually far outweigh risks from x-rays. The scan is one of the best ways of "looking" at soft tissues such as the heart and lungs.[8]

Calcium scoring is often used to identify apparently healthy individuals who are at high risk of heart attack but who do not fit the usual profile with risk factors such as obesity and smoking. Scores can range from zero to more than three thousand. Zero is often good. Three thousand is not.

Calcium scoring is still an inexact science in terms of precisely comparing scores in one individual over time, but new technology has improved accuracy greatly in the past few years.

Although calcium scores have been identified as good predictors of cardiovascular disease, *there is no apparent correlation between fitness and high or low calcium scores.*[9] This seems to run contrary to conventional wisdom about how to ward off a heart attack. One would think that a "fit" person should have a lower calcium score because such persons are supposed to be at less risk of heart disease. Yet this is often not the case. Someone who is in great shape but who has a high calcium score is at risk of heart disease. Until calcium scoring was developed, this was not known.

However, one problem with CT scans is that they don't show the fibrous cap and fats that gather around calcified deposits, so there is still an incomplete picture of blood vessel blockage.

Newer techniques, such as contrast magnetic resonance imaging (MRI) and ultrasound-enhanced CT scans, are available, and these will help to fill that gap. Another more invasive and therefore risky method is intravascular ultrasound, or IVUS. Here, a thin rod is put through the artery to help produce pictures that identify blockages and calcification. Together, such scanning techniques involve a dizzying array of technical terms, but they each show artery blockage with varying degrees of accuracy. For more descriptions on these scanning methods see the glossary.

Taken together, nanobacteria tests and calcium scoring are said to give reliable evidence of nanobacteria infections. Other tests for inflammation and clotting may give clues to the presence of nanobacteria and calcification but only in conjunction with such diagnostics.

The importance of improving these methods is high. If doctors can see and measure calcification in smaller parts of the body, then treatment may be far more effective.

Eight

Calcium Germ Exterminators

M any scientists have tried to neutralize the explosive potential of calcium deposits but usually in response to individual diseases instead of as an overall strategy. This is because calcification has been seen as *resulting from* disease rather than *triggering* it. Unfortunately, this may have been the wrong way around in many cases.

That's not to say every attempt has been ineffective. For example, citrate has been used for a few years to treat kidney stones,[1] and as we'll see, it is also an effective nanobiotic agent. But doctors didn't know that. They just saw the chemical working against the stones.

Other approaches are site-specific. Implanted heart valves that calcify have been treated with a process that modifies the local tissue to make it less susceptible to calcification.[2] Clearly this can't be used throughout the body without replacing most of what is in us.

Families of drugs known as "calcium antagonists" and "calcium channel blockers" are used to stop the pure mineral from doing nasty things to us in heart disease. It is important to not confuse these with treatments for reducing calcification. Calcium on its own plays a defining role in cell functions. Calcium antagonists and channel blockers are aimed at controlling some of these functions. Despite their widespread use, there is scant evidence that these drugs reverse calcification. Instead, there is controversy over whether the drugs are good or bad for patients who have calcification.[3] This is an important issue, but due to ambiguous and limited evidence so far, we do not cover calcium channel blockers further here.

Until now, each of these assaults on calcium and calcification has been missing one piece of basic knowledge: what triggers the deposits.

PATENTING NANOBIOTICS

By 1998, Olavi Kajander and Neva Çiftçioğlu had applied to patent formulas to eradicate nanobacteria. One of those consisted of a chemical to dissolve the calcium shell from nanobacteria and of an antibiotic or other chemical to eliminate them. The ingredients could be used in varying combinations because each had some reaction with calcium and some impacts on nanobacteria. The scientists postulated that these could get rid of calcification in illnesses such as atherosclerosis, gum disease, and kidney stones. Chemicals, including bisphosphonates that are used to treat osteoporosis, were identified in the patent.[4] Also, ampicillin, trimethoprim, and nitrofurantoin had impacts. In experiments outside the human body, chemicals that extract calcium, such as EDTA and citrate, were working.[5] Kajander was also the first to try bisphosphonates and antibiotics together on a patient for treatment of kidney stones.

It was therefore clear that more than one combination was effective. But the road from a patent or human experimentation to commercial application is rough. Government authorities have extensive mechanisms for certifying product safety. Kajander and Çiftçioğlu had started a company to commercialize their tests for detecting nanobacteria, but they and their supporters found it impossible to raise the funds for expensive treatment approval procedures. This was especially hard because the very existence of nanobacteria was still being challenged.

OTHER APPROACHES TO A PANDEMIC

Against this backdrop of regulatory and academic roadblocks, the medical community was suffering from a terrible problem that, so far, no manufactured drug had been able to beat. Around the world, millions of heart disease patients had died despite sophisticated surgery and drug treatment. The numbers were so great as to be numbing. In many cases, doctors had to bluntly tell their patients that there was nothing more to do for them and it was just a question of time before they died. Modern medicine did not have a solution for them.

To try to solve this, and while academic debates raged over nanobacteria, hundreds of medical professionals were experimenting with other chemical combinations. They were as yet unaware of Kajander and Çiftçioğlu's discovery. A procedure known as "intravenous chelation"—which we'll explore in chapter 9—was being used to try to dissolve calcium deposits in the arteries of thousands of patients. Some successes were being claimed, but there was scant published clinical evidence to support the stories.

Across the Atlantic from Kajander and Çiftçioğlu, and unknown to them at the time, one medical professional decided to apply chelating chemicals in a new way. Gary Mezo came onto the nanobacteria scene years after Kajander and Çiftçioğlu made their first discoveries. There continue to be arguments over how much original work Mezo did to improve on the researchers' active ingredients. But there is no doubt that his contribution was significant. Aside from being the first to apply a variant of the nanobiotic treatment for heart disease patients, his main role was to bring immediate benefits to patients who had exhausted every other alternative.

To do this he took some calculated risks.

THE ETHICAL DILEMMA

His use of an ages-old loophole, discussed later in this chapter, sparked controversy in the regulatory and research communities because at that time no clinical studies had been done on the treatment. However, weighing against this criticism was the reality that millions of heart patients were dying after modern medicine had done everything to save them.

This typified a dilemma confronting every cardiologist every day: send patients home to die, or risk a new treatment that has not gone through exhaustive clinical trial? Part of that predicament involves relative risk: the severity and stage of the disease compared to the positive and negative results that have been observed with an experimental treatment.

Many patients know about that dilemma because there had been a loud argument about it over treatments for AIDS and cancer. Ironically though, while the discussion has been loudest with those diseases, far more patients die from heart disease.

Gary Mezo decided that, given the balance of risks and benefits that he perceived and the opinions of physicians whom he consulted with, it was worthwhile to suggest to doctors that they go ahead with a revolutionary approach. Eventually, this would come to be known as "nanobiotics," although the term had also been applied to other unrelated treatments.

WHERE CONVENTIONAL AND ALTERNATIVE MEET

Mezo's approach combined conventional and alternative medicine. He began his medical studies like every other student—in physiology and premedicine—but said that finances intervened and he had to step sideways by starting with nurse practitioner (N.P.) and physician's assistant (P.A.) degrees.

Today, most patients in the United States are seen by an N.P. or P.A. at one time or another. They diagnose, treat, prescribe medicines, deliver babies in a pinch, and do much of what M.D.s do. It is now commonly accepted for N.P.s and P.A.s to serve as primary care providers instead of an M.D.[6] It's no exaggeration to say that many medical establishments would not function effectively without N.P.s and P.A.s.

Mezo began to see increasing numbers of patients who were taking nutritional supplements—now known as "nutraceuticals"[7]—and herbal medicines. Although these were classified as over-the-counter products, he suspected that they were having profound effects and interactions with conventional medicines. But he did not then have the physiology or pharmacology background to understand the interplay because conventional medical training did not routinely include naturopathic studies. He wasn't alone. Many medical professionals had only a limited background in nutritional supplements.

The nutraceutical groundswell had started with vitamins, moved on to supplements for memory, and finally escalated to herbal remedies for applications such as cholesterol reduction. Mezo noted that many patients were improving with some of these alternatives.

Most importantly, drugs developed by the pharmaceutical industry were often taken from herbal sources, then synthesized, renamed, and repackaged. Ironically, while herbalists were derided in conventional medicine, drug companies extracted ingredients from the same herbs that herbalists used, then marketed them profitably.

Like others, Mezo saw that patients died despite surgery and drugs designed to control their heart disease. None of these approaches was reversing the core atherosclerosis and few if any treatments were getting rid of the accompanying inflammation.

That widespread failure spurred Mezo to study naturopathy to understand the chemical relationships between herbal and conventional drugs. According to him, one day a patient in his forties who'd had a heart attack came to Mezo's Tampa office in tears. A short time before his attack, he'd led a vibrant, active life. Afterward though, he'd been off work for months and his finances were in ruins. He desperately asked Mezo why no one could help him despite billions of dollars spent on heart disease.

The alternative medicine world was using a type of chelation that removes heavy metals from blood. (Chelation's extensive and controversial history[8] is summarized in chapter 9.) Mezo perceived that chelation wasn't working in heart disease as proponents said it should. Claims about how its pharmacological mechanisms functioned made no sense to him. Many patients appeared to get better briefly, but then they generally relapsed some time after treatment. Also, the treatment was time-consuming and expensive. Because it was administered intravenously it required a visit to a doctor's office several times a week for three or four hours.

Yet at least one chemical used in chelation, EDTA (ethylenediamine-tetraacetic acid), appeared to consistently show temporary benefits.[9] This chemical also "sequesters," or sucks out, harmful calcium deposits.

With the forty-year-old patient in mind, Mezo began to scrutinize conventional and alternative heart drug therapies. He concluded that most were administered in the wrong place at the wrong time of day and were missing ingredients that might help to dissolve calcified plaque.

THE FIRST STEPS

He devised a formula that could be administered at home by patients. It included amino acids and enzyme systems that he thought would help to promote the opening of veins and arteries along with removal of calcium deposits from atherosclerotic plaque.

He substituted a suppository for intravenous use of EDTA. He was convinced that, if it were used on a daily basis, it would be safe and physiologically effective.

Mezo's experience and study suggested to him that EDTA would not irritate the rectum and would be absorbed into the blood like other drugs administered by suppository. Digestive functions can destroy the effectiveness of many drugs, but rectal insertion lets them bypass the stomach and intestines, reducing the amount of drug required.

He then had a pharmacist "compound" the preparation. Without compounding, this treatment may have never made it to so many patients as early as it did, so it's worthwhile to look at the role that this ancient art plays in medicine.

Compounding is as old as the civilized world. It involves putting together chemical ingredients to make a treatment for a patient. All pharmacists are trained as chemists or apothecaries to do this.

Some pharmacists still mix ingredients for individual patients but Americans don't hear much about this because most drugs are manufactured by large companies. Compounding is essential for prescriptions that suit the specific needs of patients, because some treatments are used too seldom to be profitably manufactured by drug companies, while other compounds must match the dosage requirements of each patient.

Compounding has been dying out in America and parts of Europe over the past seventy years. However, the trend has been far from uniform. In Italy, for example, compounding has remained more prevalent. In emerging economies such as China's, it retains a pervasive presence. Also, the practice has been making a comeback in postindustrial economies since the late 1990s due to new demands from physicians and patients for customized treatments. Now, thousands of compounded prescriptions are prepared daily.

A thin legal line separates compounding from more heavily regulated manufacturing. Compounders and American regulators have often locked horns on who has the right to do what. According to American legislation, pharmacists who compound are exempt from being regulated as manufacturers if the drug product is

> compounded for an identified individual patient based on the unsolicited receipt of a valid prescription order or a notation, approved by the prescribing practitioner, on the prescription order that a compounded product is necessary for the identified patient (21 USC §353a(a)).[10]

In plain English, this means that a physician must write a prescription for the patient and deliver it to a pharmacist. Then the pharmacist compounds the prescription for that individual patient. According to American regulatory agencies' interpretation of the law, drug companies have to stay out of the physician-patient-pharmacist triangle for compounding to be legal. A company can license a product to a pharmacy, but it cannot be involved in advising doctors or patients on its use. That falls to pharmacists.

Manufacturing, on the other hand, involves producing doses by the millions, packaging them, and reselling them to pharmacies. Here, drug companies are actively involved in marketing the product to physicians and patients. This only involves the pharmacist when he or she takes some premanufactured doses out of a bottle and puts them into a smaller bottle for a patient.

EXPERIMENTATION

Mezo used a certain interpretation of regulations governing compounding to bring his treatment to patients without going through a multiyear approval process that is required for manufactured drugs. He designed a prescription compound of established generic medicines, using suppositories and a powder that extended the time frame for EDTA to work in the blood.

According to him, he then did something that many doctors do but won't admit to: he tried the medication on himself. When he saw that there were no apparent ill effects, he began working with four cardiac patients who faced probable death from their illness. They had an incentive to try a new approach.

To his delight, patients who had been "cardiac cripples" appeared to improve. They were walking without chest pain and reported positive side effects such as better eyesight. A few men said that their erectile function was enhanced.

These were only preliminary and sometimes anecdotal results. Mezo was worried about kidney function because EDTA is reported to cause stress on the kidneys.[11] However, he says that the clinical measurements he took, along with observed kidney function, began to improve in each patient.[12] Liver function also indicated improvement. Therefore, he perceived that safety was not an immediate problem, especially considering the dire position of these last-ditch patients.

Despite this success, his results were incomplete. They suggested that the decalcification of blood vessels was only proceeding to a certain point. Something was preventing them from improving further.

CUTTING THROUGH THE RED TAPE

One night his computer mouse led him to an obscure Finnish Web site named "Nanobac Oy." It was the site of the diagnostics company that Kajander, Çiftçioğlu, and some investors had started years earlier. Mezo, who says that until then he had no idea that nanobacteria existed, saw the missing link between his treatment and their discovery of how to eradicate nanobacteria. The way that they were preparing the nanobacteria was to pour EDTA on them to dissolve their calcium shells. That suggested why EDTA was working in patients. It appeared to be dissolving the calcified shell that encased nanobacteria.

By then Kajander and Çiftçioğlu had also published their discovery that an antibiotic such as tetracycline could eradicate nanobacteria once the shells were dissolved. Reading about the tetracycline-nanobacteria connection made Mezo see how his nanobiotic therapy could be improved.[13]

Mezo also learned that Kajander and Çiftçioğlu, in collaboration with László Puskás from the Hungarian Academy of Sciences, had isolated the nanobacteria in atherosclerotic plaque.

The requirement to simultaneously dissolve the calcified armor and eliminate the nanobacteria explained why therapies that didn't do both were succeeding only temporarily to improve the conditions of heart patients before they started to get worse again. Nanobacteria were being exposed, and some were being excreted, but the rest were unleashed to cause havoc.

After many tries Mezo finally got Neva Çiftçioğlu on the telephone. She was skeptical and says that she didn't believe his story about treating patients with a method similar to one that they had been using in the lab. If true, it would catapult implementation years ahead.

After a few more discussions, Mezo was on a plane to Kuopio, Finland.

Kajander and Çiftçioğlu were astonished to find that Mezo had circumnavigated years of what would have been regulatory red tape for them in Europe by using ingredients that were individually approved by authorities and compounded as a prescription, thus, he said, avoiding the need for regulatory approval. But that was only part of why he had been able to apply the treatment quickly. Additionally, millions were suffering from a terminal condition—end-stage atherosclerosis—for which there was no cure. They urgently needed a solution.

It didn't take long for the two sides to realize that collaboration might accelerate treatment by years and save or enhance thousands, if not millions, of lives.

By 2002, less than two years after the experimental therapy had first been tried, physicians were noticing that heart patients treated with the therapy were doing something unusual. They were not dying. On top of that, they were improving. Thus, a stark contrast emerged between scientists' disbelief about nanobacteria and measurable evidence that coronary artery disease indicators were being reversed.

Throughout history, medical professionals had treated patients with compounds whose effectiveness was only later deciphered by science. In this case, though, it was not an untested "home remedy" that was being used. Patients were given well-known chemicals that had been prescribed for decades *but not in this combination.*

A SHIFT TO A NUTRITIONAL SUPPLEMENT

By 2004, a new development had broadened accessibility of the product. To get around what was becoming an increasingly contentious discussion with American regulatory authorities over the fine line between compounding and manufacturing, the company that controlled the nanobiotic separated the nondrug component and licensed the rest as a manufactured nutritional supplement.

The main advantage was that the supplement could be made in large batches and sold over-the-counter in various countries. Another plus for doctors and patients was that the ingredients were listed on the label, so there was more transparency about the treatment.

The disadvantage was that the drug part of the treatment—antibiotics—had to be prescribed separately by a physician. The other disadvantage for the company was that those who sell nutraceuticals are more strictly prohibited by U.S. law from making claims about their disease-treating properties; therefore, the properties of the treatment would now have to be relayed to patients by their doctors, not the developers. Furthermore, nutritional supplements had been coming under pressure to be more closely regulated, and despite vociferous objections from users of such supplements, there was a risk that the government might begin demanding expensive certification for that class of substances.

In view of all this, representatives of the company that controlled the nanobiotic formula took the position that the nutritional supplement was an important but still short-term step in the effort to eradicate nanobacteria. Their research was broadening into everything from vaccines to ways of getting around suppositories. While they did that, the original formula was there for patients to use immediately.

SCIENCE MEETS COMMERCE

Early on, Mezo had insisted on a close commercial relationship with Kajander and Çiftçioğlu to lock in the intellectual property. World markets had just endured one of the worst meltdowns for technology companies during a crash that began in 2000. This made capital financing difficult to get, therefore Mezo argued that combining their resources made sense.

Yet by 2003, those same difficulties in getting capital funding led Mezo's company to merge with another corporation that was trading as a publicly owned firm in American markets. That brought new management into the equation. Ironically, as with so many start-ups in the brutal entrepreneurial cycle, the founder had to step aside to make way for new commercial and managerial realities.

The significance was that nanobiotics went from being developed in a privately controlled and managed enterprise to being part of a publicly scrutinized one. The move invited yet more attention from regulators. The discussion over compounding of products grew more intensive, leading to the earlier-described reformulation, along with licensing of distribution to yet another company.

What had begun as a halting struggle by a few individuals was blossoming into a multinational race to decipher and commercially exploit the secrets of nanobacteria. The first part of that story belonged to the Europeans. Discoveries about human nanobacteria had started with a Finnish physician studying in America, a Turkish microbiologist who found her way to Finland and then Houston, and a Hungarian researcher who isolated the organisms in arterial plaque. The work had then expanded to include American and British researchers and an American medical entrepreneur, who, while developing a prescription compound, crossed paths with the Europeans. The role of the Americans subsequently grew more prominent on the business side. At least one publicly traded company was commercializing nanobacteria discoveries. Finally, as in so many areas, the role of Asia grew suddenly significant. Researchers in China and South Korea began publishing groundbreaking work on nanobacteria. In 2004, the Sino-Finland Nanobacteria Co-Operation Center was inaugurated at Central South University in Changsha, Hunan province, China.[14]

At the core of that globalized competition and cooperation was the work of Kajander and Çiftçioğlu, combined with the entrepreneurial approach of American medical experts. The varying cultures, temperaments, genders, scientific philosophies, and religious views of these players made a rich and volatile mix. Their lives intersected at the point where research, commerce, and the treatment of desperately ill patients met. This confluence led to clashes on more than one occasion. Amid the changes, Çiftçioğlu and Kajander remained ambivalent about commercialization. As research scientists, they prized their academic freedom. Çiftçioğlu in particular was focused on the nonprofit aspects of research and said she was not interested in deriving commercial benefits, although she had been a shareholder in the original Finnish company that was selling tests for detecting nanobacteria. Her personal focus remained research. As testament to that, in 2002 she began collaborating with the American space agency NASA on research into nanobacteria in astronauts and the possibility that it might be found as a life form on other planets. Kajander, on the other hand, elected to get involved with research under the umbrella of a corporation while maintaining his academic research position in Finland.

From these events, one thing was certain; the tension between free scientific inquiry and commercial exploitation remained. As work on nanobacteria progressed, compromises between "open source" research and intellectual property protection would play a defining role. The outcome had the potential to influence the lives of a generation of patients.

Nine
Reversing a Slow-Motion Blast

A t least one treatment aimed at eradicating human nanobacteria has been developed and tried.[1] According to its inventors it has been used with thousands of patients who have heart disease or are at high risk. After several years' experience, the nanobiotic was reformulated to make it more broadly available, but its developers said that the ingredients were largely the same as the original ones.

Here we look at that formula to see how it works. This is only an early step in what will ultimately be varying approaches as research into nanobiotics accelerates.

For heart disease, here again are the main components that a treatment must address: First and foremost is inflammation that makes vessel walls swell. Accompanying that is plaque that coats blood vessels and is composed of a messy, complex mix of fats (cholesterol and other lipids), calcium deposits, a fibrous cap, and globules of other organic materials. Then there is clotting that attempts to quell the perceived injuries. Often these components conspire to cause tiny blockages that doctors may not notice at first. A series of slow-motion events leads up to a catastrophic blast in the body. It is not easy to just clean out this mess and reverse the effects in a short time.

A REMINDER OF TOXICITY

Remember that calcium phosphate particles are not just inconvenient. They can wreak havoc when they come in contact with cells. They have been shown to cause swelling and make cells replicate rapidly. They are not just another inactive component of heart disease; they are ongoing irritants that assault us continuously.

Nanobacteria researchers emphasize this toxicity because critics often portray calcification as an effect instead of a cause. By so doing they overlook a catalyst that requires treatment on its own. Getting rid of the trigger for calcification is not just relieving a symptom, it is removing an insidious threat to arterial health.

With that in mind, let's look at steps used in the original treatment to address this.

THREE STEPS

The treatment has been administered at home once a day by the patient in three parts (a suppository, an antibiotic capsule, and a nutraceutical that was once dissolved in a liquid but then later put into capsule form):

▣ The suppository contained a base with the calcium dissolving and removing agent EDTA.

▣ The capsule contained tetracycline hydrochloride (commonly abbreviated as tetracycline), an antibiotic that is effective against nanobacteria.

▣ The nutraceutical contained enzymes and amino acid systems to dissolve fibrolipid deposits and soft plaque. It also sustained levels of disodium calcium EDTA to dissolve calcified deposits. The 2004 label of the product displayed a proprietary blend of vitamins, minerals, amino acids, and enzymes including EDTA, vitamin C, L-arginine, L-lysine, L-ornithine, vitamin B_6, bromelain, trypsin, niacin, CoQ_{10}, grapeseed extract, hawthorn berry, papain, folic acid, and selenium.[2]

According to the product's developers, to dissolve atherosclerotic plaque and to get rid of nanobacteria in various stages of development, these three components have to be used together as indicated by a qualified physician.

EDTA

The colorless organic compound EDTA is used to bind and extract heavy metals. It is approved by the FDA as a safe food additive.[3] The food industry uses thousands of tons of it to prevent decomposition of food by trace metals, such as copper, iron, and nickel, that catalyze the oxidation of fats and cause food to get rancid. EDTA is an all-purpose ingredient. It is used in detergents, liquid soaps, shampoos, agricultural chemical sprays, pharmaceutical products, oil emulsions, and textiles to do everything from improving dyeing to enhancing scouring and detergent operations.[4]

For many years EDTA has also been used in chelation therapy to remove heavy metals from the body and in attempts to dissolve calcification of the arteries. Since there is a wealth of contradictory information in medical journals and from medical practitioners about chelation, it's important to distinguish between the nanobiotic application of EDTA and chelation as it is usually practiced.

The term "chelation" stems from the Greek word *chele*, meaning "claw," for chemicals that grab metal particles such as aluminum, lead, mercury, and cadmium and minerals such as calcium. Once in the blood, EDTA binds to these elements. The resulting combination is excreted from the body during urination.[5] In this way, chelation has been used as the preferred treatment for lead poisoning for more than fifty years.[6]

Some physicians say that there are also potential benefits for coronary artery disease.[7] However, they add that these advantages should not be confused with questionable claims about the effects on calcification in atherosclerosis. For example, as early as the 1950s it was hypothesized that EDTA could get rid of calcification in arterial plaque, but this is still a controversial claim.[8] Some chelation therapists maintain that their methods reduce calcification of the arteries.[9] Yet clinical studies have not shown sustainable, statistically significant decreases in atherosclerotic calcification. One trial of intravenous use of EDTA (administered by injection) claimed to show no measurable benefits for coronary artery disease patients.[10] However, that study too has been criticized for its methods,[11] so the situation remains confusing.

Most medical associations are skeptical and say that clinical proof of intravenous chelation's effectiveness is lacking.[12] But the National Institutes of Health (NIH) has not yet discounted its potential value. At the time of writing, a $30 million NIH study was attempting to answer the question more definitively.[13]

The NIH has summarized the various theories by chelation proponents about EDTA. It might directly remove calcium from fatty plaques that block arteries, causing the plaques to disintegrate. Or it may stimulate the release of a hormone that causes calcium to be removed from plaques. The therapy may reduce damaging effects of oxygen ions on the walls of blood vessels. This might reduce inflammation and improve blood vessel function. However, the NIH concludes, "None of these theories has been well tested in scientific studies."[14]

The claim that calcification can be reduced by combining intravenous chelation with oral tetracycline has also been criticized. While there is a lack of scientific study to prove this one way or the other, here is how the critique goes:[15]

The half-life of serum EDTA for intravenous use is short, so the chemical is excreted through the kidneys quickly. Intravenous EDTA is also given when the patient is awake, so the metabolic rate is high and clearance is rapid. If you've just eaten, you'll have a high load of free metabolic ions in the bloodstream from digestion. The chemical processes in the body (metabolic rate), together with other changes generated by digesting food, is thought to reduce the effects of EDTA. Furthermore, it is argued that EDTA suppositories combined with tetracycline at bedtime do not work any more effectively than intravenous EDTA because this method doesn't maintain adequate serum levels. Another component is required to do that.

Some chelation proponents disagree with these arguments, but in the absence of clinical trial comparisons it is hard to tell who is right.

Here are differences that have been said to distinguish the nanobiotic approach from what is commonly referred to as "chelation therapy":

- Most chelation requires a patient to visit the doctor's office several times a week for an expensive, time-consuming, and uncomfortable intravenous procedure, whereas nanobiotics are self-administered at home, eliminating medical visits that interfere with lifestyle and work.

- Conventional chelation "unroofs" nanobacteria but may not get rid of them. Without using integrated therapies to neutralize them, the risks of unroofing nanobacteria from their dormant state are high. They may cause trouble—including risk of heart attacks—when they get loose in the blood. That may explain, for example, why many patients appear to get temporarily better with intravenous chelation, then get worse. The phenomenon is not limited to chelation. Patients who've had kidney stones pulverized or stents put into their arteries also have relapses. Such conditions may share the same cause: unroofed nanobacteria plant themselves as "seeds" from which new growths develop. The nanobiotic therapy targets those nanobacteria, whereas administration of EDTA alone does not.

◙ With the nanobiotic method, EDTA is not administered at the same time of day or in the same way as with conventional chelation. Instead, the nanobiotic approach leads to fundamental differences in the way that the body metabolizes EDTA.

Other physicians agree that this particular combination of EDTA with ingredients and protocols is special, but they add that whether it is or isn't chelation is a question of semantics.[16] They point out that chelating chemicals are still part of the therapy.

Dr. James Roberts, who administered the original nanobiotic, also emphasizes that not one death related to chelation therapy has been reported to the Food and Drug Administration. Therefore, he believes that the claim about its other risks is overblown.[17]

The fact that EDTA removes heavy metals such as lead is not essential to get at nanobacteria, but some say that it may help to detoxify patients, thus enhancing the treatment's effects. As explained earlier, there is clinical evidence of such detoxification.[18]

A suppository method of delivering EDTA was developed and patented in the mid-1990s.[19] The chemical is contained in a glycerin-type material that melts gradually in the rectum and is absorbed into the blood. The EDTA is also bound in a controlled-release form so that it takes several hours to have its full effects.

Most Europeans have few compunctions about suppositories, but many Americans have a phobia about them. The first reaction of some American patients is "Yuck! I'm not gonna do that!"

However, for seriously ill patients, the choice is stark: do or die. Furthermore, a suppository is much less discomforting and dangerous than undergoing coronary bypass surgery or being on heart drugs for the rest of their lives.

TETRACYCLINE

Then we see another revolution: using an old gun to fight a new enemy. Tetracycline has been used for decades to fight many infections but fell into disuse for many applications. This was due to resistance by bacteria and—some argue—to the expiration of patents that makes the drug unprofitable for drug companies.

According to Nanobac Life Sciences, which at the time of writing controlled the patents for the treatment, tetracycline may be effective because nanobacteria do not yet seem to be resistant to the drug. It is theorized that once the fibrous cap is dissipated and the calcium has been dissolved, the semidormant particles are vulnerable. Yet these "encased" nanobacteria aren't the only ones in the human body. Other, younger ones that haven't yet encased themselves are actively emitting toxic biofilm. When tetracycline is administered, it immediately begins to get rid of the unencased free-roaming nanobacteria while attacking the encased ones that have just been exposed by EDTA.

Other antibiotics neutralize the infection but only if the drugs are administered at levels that are toxic to humans.[20] Still others work without being toxic but don't work as well. Tetracycline seems to have fewer side effects and the highest effectiveness.[21]

One side effect may also make tetracycline the antibiotic of choice. It *binds well with calcium*.[22] This has often been seen as a drawback because it leads to yellowing of teeth in children. Yet researchers theorize that for older adults it may help to strip the defensive calcium coating off the nanobacteria and prevent the coating from reforming.

THE NUTRACEUTICAL COMPONENT

The EDTA-tetracycline combination is said to be enhanced by a third group of ingredients contained in a nutritional supplement. According to a company Web page that describes the treatment, the supplement

> consists of essential amino acids, enzymes, antioxidants and natural anti-inflammatory components. The overall purpose . . . is to reduce and remove soft fibrous fatty plaque, which is the majority of overall plaque volume.[23]

The Web page description adds that the supplement's components help to boost the immune system and mitigate other conditions:

> The first improvement many people notice . . . is a decrease in symptoms of arthritis due to the regimen's natural anti-inflammatory components. Additionally, many people see improvements in lipid levels (cholesterol), blood glucose levels (sugar levels) in diabetics and marked improvements in angina symptoms.[24]

A quick tour of the Internet or the supplements aisle of a health food store shows that numerous ingredients in the nutritional supplement are also in other heart-related products. These are aimed at improving the elasticity of arteries, lowering cholesterol, thinning blood, removing plaque, and repairing injury. For details on these ingredients and what they are designed to do, please refer to the glossary.

Critics and supporters point out that so far the impacts of such components have not been quantified in this particular treatment. For example, vitamin C, niacin (vitamin B_3), and bromelain are shown in medical literature to have fibrinogen-reducing properties. Fibrinogen is found in the fibrotic cap of atherosclerotic plaque, and must be removed so that other chemicals can get at the underlying plaque. Studies have been done on such ingredients individually and impacts have been measured. Still, the area remains greatly understudied by conventional medical authorities.

This is not to say that such ingredients are ineffective but instead that Western medical science has only begun to seriously examine the physiological effects of nutraceuticals on heart disease. In the United States, the National Institutes of Health have just started to finance research into this area. Renowned universities such as the University of California, Los Angeles have initiated institutes in the field. The Europeans seem further advanced. However, in China, administration of nutritional supplements has been practiced and studied for decades.

THE RIGHT COMBINATION AND "COMPLIANCE"

Once the treatment is administered, a war begins in the human body as years of stealthy buildup begin to come undone. In test-tube experiments it has been shown that nanobacteria "unroofed" by EDTA come out of their dormant stage, secrete biofilm, and begin to clump together to defend themselves. This can cause trouble for cardiac patients if the special nanobiotic sequence is not applied. Too much clumping of nanobacteria may precipitate clotting and lead to a heart attack. Therefore, physicians have emphasized that it is important to use the three weapons together precisely as they were designed: the nutraceutical component to help deal with coronary risk factors such as inflammation and toxins, EDTA suppositories to break the shells around nanobacteria, and tetracycline to fight the nanobacteria themselves. And patients have to stick with the regimen for anywhere from four months to more than a year. Physicians also recommend that patients continue using their present heart drugs until their doctor says that it is safe to reduce their frequency or use.

Poor compliance is a major issue in medicine. Studies show that many patients don't take their drugs long or often enough or at the right time and that this is responsible for up to 125,000 deaths per year in the United States alone from cardiovascular disease.[25] That is about three times the annual death toll from car accidents in America.

Is occasional noncompliance harmful to the nanobiotic treatment? According to the developers, accidentally missing a day or two doesn't seem to be crucial as long as the treatment is restarted and then continued as prescribed. However, this remains to be confirmed in clinical studies.

SWITCHING FROM COMPOUND TO NUTRACEUTICAL

The compounded prescription has been divided into a manufactured nutritional supplement available over the counter and an antibiotic prescribed by a physician. Has this reformulation altered the basic treatment? According to the company that licenses the product, no. The only difference aside from breaking out the tetracycline was to put the nutraceutical into capsule form to make it more palatable.

The shift from formulating a compound to manufacturing a nutritional supplement may seem minor, but from regulatory and availability viewpoints it may be profound. Aside from implications for the American markets, many other countries allow the importation of nutritional supplements more readily than compounded drugs. The listing of ingredients on the label may also open the product to more competition, although competitors will still have to deal with legal considerations surrounding the patented combination of EDTA and antibiotics.

Will compounding continue to hold importance for nanobiotics? According to researchers who work with it, yes, especially in countries where nutritional supplements and antibiotics can be compounded without running afoul of regulatory requirements. This may hold true especially in developing nations.

Yet the real question is, does the treatment produce measurable results when used against heart disease or other illnesses?

Ten

What Doctors and Patients Discovered

With early nanobiotics there has been a classic contrast between physicians who say "It works for my patients" and skeptics who say "Prove it."

What is acceptable evidence that a treatment works? The first is laboratory proof of what eradicates an infection outside the body, based on papers published in peer-reviewed journals. This has been done repeatedly for nanobacteria. The next, as we'll see here, is clinical measurements taken by physicians of their patients' conditions prior to and after treatment for an infection. Such measurements are based on direct observation of a patient by a qualified physician. Objective clinical data are different from hearsay or anecdotal evidence such as "I feel better." Clinical data include quantifiable measurements of blood and other factors. These are explained further in the glossary, under the term "clinical evidence."

Then there is a clinical trial monitored by an independent review board. We'll examine one trial here.

Finally there is anecdotal evidence: statements by patients about their experiences and by physicians about the general state of their patients' health. Whether this is "acceptable" is the topic of many debates.

Taken alone, each form of evidence is convincing but incomplete. Critics claim the pieces are too scattered to draw definite conclusions from. Yet together, those clues tell a compelling story.

FOR PATIENTS WITHOUT OTHER OPTIONS

Early nanobiotics have been at the core of risk-benefit debates over applying experimental treatments to gravely ill patients. Some experts say that such treatments should not be administered without exhaustive clinical trials. On the other hand, the ethical questions are these: With patients who have nothing left to lose, is it acceptable to withhold a treatment with well-known ingredients that has shown promising preliminary results? Whose place is it to allow patients to die without recourse to such experimental therapies?

Because millions of seriously ill heart patients have exhausted other treatments, advocate physicians argue that it is more responsible to proceed cautiously than to wait. These patients are considered "too far gone" by most physicians to be saved from a slow decline to the grave. They have used up their available surgical, drug, and "alternative" options. Exploring new possibilities for this group was a driving motivation for these doctors. On one hand, they did not want to offer false hope or to claim that scientific proof exists where it doesn't. On the other hand, experience with this approach suggested that using well-known ingredients in new ways might help such patients.

These physicians do not claim that all applications of this therapy have been successful with critically ill patients. However, they *do* claim that every patient has a right to know and decide, instead of being denied the right to make a decision.

They also emphasize that the merits of this experimental therapy have to be compared to the seriousness of a patient's condition. The treatment was initially developed for the most ill cardiac patients. For such patients, not dying is remarkable on its own.

These excerpts from subjective testimonials by patients are examples of what was reported so far. As we'll see, they are far from being the only evidence of results.

Patient with classic atherosclerosis symptoms:

> [T]he turnaround in my health situation has been nothing short of miraculous.

> Last August, I was having some serious problems including difficulty breathing, chest pains, a rapid heart beat, lack of energy and overall, a very down feeling.

> Within six weeks after commencing the treatment, I improved dramatically and these problems resolved. I no longer have difficulty breath-

ing, chest pains, walking distances and I am once again, positive and enthusiastic. I now feel that I have stopped aging.

. . . My initial spiral heart [CT] scan test done on September 6, 2001, [shows] a total calcification score of 451.7 and my second test on December 18, 2001, [shows] a total score of 348. This is a drop of 103.7 points in three and a half months, which to me is astounding.[1]

Heart patient with urinary problems:

Prior to treatment: Tired, sleepy, urinated about every 3–4 hours day and night, partial loss of bladder control, irritability. Swollen feet. Abnormal heart rhythm. Calcium score of 3700.

After treatment: Felt stronger, more alert, don't seem to need over seven hours sleep. Urinate less often and have more control over bladder. Less audible heart rhythm. Less edema. Feet and legs less swollen. Observable improvements after 6–8 months. Calcium score after eight months reduced to 1700. Has been in treatment for 13 months.

Heart patient with angina:

Prior to treatment: Angina. Had stents inserted after clot in heart. OK for eight or so months then angina recurred. Started to fall down for no apparent reason. Was classified as an "eleventh hour" case and recommended for open-heart surgery. Did not do that but started nanobiotic treatment.

After treatment: Angina essentially gone. Ten minutes on treadmill, no angina. Blood pressure generally lower. Feel better overall. Better stamina. Treatment reduced to 2 weeks on, 2 weeks off. Lost 25 pounds. Discontinued some heart drugs. Stopped nitroglycerine use. Mood has improved. Side effects: looser bowels.

Dermatology patient with chronic rashes:

Prior to treatment. For more than 20 years had skin rashes. Dermatologists prescribed creams. They would work for a short time then another rash came. Had rash all over body that "itched and itched."

After treatment. After first month of treatment noticed improvement. After three months, was free of rash. Then cut down treatment to three times a week, then two. Then stopped all treatment. Then the rashes started again. Took treatment for 16 days and it cleared up. Now takes three treatments at the beginning of each month. Gums are in better shape.

At first had some diarrhea and flatulence but that went away.[2]

Heart patient who is an M.D. allergist:

> Before treatment: Intense jaw and neck pain while exercising. Obstruction
> of right coronary artery. Couldn't walk up two flights of stairs "without
> getting in trouble." Stent was put in but then blocked.

> After treatment: Calcium score dropped by at least 25 percent. Pain
> gone during exercise. Dropped back treatment to two weeks per month,
> then stopped, but continues with his regularly prescribed heart drugs. No
> negative side effects. A cataract in his eye has disappeared.

> "If this is as good as it looks on paper right now and [knowing that] I'm
> feeling as good as I have felt in the past year and a half, for example
> my stent should have plugged over and it hasn't . . . I just have to think
> that there has to be something going on that's a positive situation at
> least for me."[3]

THE MARATHON CARDIOLOGIST

Dr. James C. Roberts practices what he preaches by maintaining a rigorous exercise regimen. He runs about forty miles a week. Such determina-
tion may explain why he is one of the few mainstream cardiologists who
has successfully treated patients with what was once seen as an alternative
therapy known as "enhanced external counter pulsation" (EECP).

EECP is a good example of a therapy that relieves heart disease symptoms for very ill patients and improves their chances for avoiding a heart
attack but does not cure the disease. With this therapy, pneumatic cuffs
are placed over the patient's lower extremities, then inflated and deflated
repeatedly. This drives oxygenated blood backward from the lower parts
of the body into the heart. That, in turn, increases pressure between the
open arteries and those blocked by heart disease. The pressure stimulates
formation of small natural "bypasses." That is, the body expands its own
tiny arteries. The therapy is used often for patients who are considered to
be "too far gone" to undergo stent implants or bypass surgery.

According to Roberts, EECP is a low-risk, noninvasive procedure that
can be done quickly outside the hospital. A full course of therapy typically
involves thirty-five one-hour treatments done over seven weeks. The cost
is a fraction of that for bypass surgery or angioplasty. EECP is covered by
most commercial insurers, the major health maintenance organizations
that serve Roberts's local area, and government Medicare.[4]

Roberts is the medical director of the EECP Center of Toledo, Ohio.
He has about two decades of experience in cardiology. He doesn't like
losing patients, especially to premature death. Yet in his practice, where

the worst cardiac cases end up, it's a brutal fact of life. That's why he started looking at therapies outside conventional ones that were only of limited use to his patients.

Since 1997 he had successfully used EECP with hundreds of patients. Yet he still faced a problem. It was far more difficult to successfully apply EECP if patients had advanced blockage in their lower extremities, didn't have one good artery left from which to grow natural bypasses, or suffered from irregular heartbeat (arrhythmia) or heart failure.

"Unfortunately," Roberts laments, "half of the patients referred to us by other cardiologists have one of these four complicating features. Now we can stabilize the cardiac rhythm with drugs, and heart failure can be compensated for medically, but if all three arteries of the heart are blocked, or if there is poor blood flow to the legs—well, then we're stuck. We can try as hard as we can and the patient can try as hard as he/she can, but these patients don't get a good result. This is upsetting, as to these patients, EECP was their 'last hope.'"[5]

Many patients were suffering and dying—a sad but not unusual phenomenon in end-stage heart disease victims.

Then in May 2001 Roberts came across the work of Gary Mezo, who theorized, based on a pilot study, that arterial blockage results from long-standing infection by an organism that can be treated. Roberts says that initially, "I got a good laugh at Mezo's expense—what a ridiculous theory. I 'knew' that atherosclerosis was due to high cholesterol and the other risk factors that we 'knew' about."

But Mezo claimed in his pilot study that when ninety patients were treated, their calcium scores fell.[6] These scores, taken from rapid x-rays of the arteries, measure dangerous calcium buildups that can trigger heart attacks (see the glossary for details on calcium scoring).

Roberts was experiencing what other physicians across America were going through—a disbelieving but fascinated reaction to what appeared to be a crazy claim: coronary calcification was being reversed.

Like other doctors, he also had to overcome a deep discomfort with prescribing a drug whose contents he was not totally aware of. Ingredients of the nutraceutical component were a trade secret at the time, although that has since changed as we saw in chapter 9. He also wasn't happy with what he saw as some overly optimistic claims by the treatment's developers.

Yet the alternatives—continued pain and certain death among his patients—drove him to tell them about the treatment and suggest that they try it.

Discoveries from observation of patients

Roberts was among the first to discover that the clinical signs in patients started to improve. They didn't just improve slightly; they improved remarkably. For example, some patients who had no pulse in their feet due to arterial blockage started to have one again. Most cardiologists had never seen such a restoration of pulse. It signified that something profound was going on.

He made another important discovery: in some cases, calcium scores didn't change in the first course of treatment, but patients still exhibited clinical signs of improvement. They also started to feel better prior to significant reductions in their calcification levels. Calcification is the toughest component to get rid of compared to inflammation, clotting, and soft plaque in atherosclerosis. Thus, while calcification may be triggering the problem, it is also one of the last measurable heart disease indicators to be reversed. According to other researchers and physicians who work with nanobiotics, this is why patients first begin to show improvements in their blood and in signs of inflammation. Then only later do physical indicators of calcification reduction begin to show. This may help to explain why some of the first improvements are seen in patients' general energy levels long before their calcium scores start to drop.

Roberts made such landmark observations about nanobiotics in case histories that he published on his Web site.[7] The results include heart scan images that show calcium reduction, plus other results that clinically demonstrate improved cardiovascular function.

Following are excerpts from those case histories.

(Note: Some of the material in these pages is more technical than in the rest of this book because it describes clinical evidence that has been observed by a practicing physician. Such observations are included here so that patients and physicians can get a more complete picture. Selected passages are paraphrased and in some parts taken from Roberts's reports and correspondence.)[8]

Patient MP: *atherosclerosis everywhere*

MP had severe vascular disease. In 1992 she underwent bypass surgery on several arteries, followed by multidrug treatment. That went on until 2001, when she began to experience chest pains once or twice daily. She suffered from severe blockage of the arteries in her lower extremities and had no pulse in her feet. She also had a kidney cyst and narrowing in the arteries to the kidneys, brain, and left arm. She had atherosclerosis everywhere and wasn't a candidate for further medical procedures. With her severe disease, she also wasn't a candidate for EECP (a treatment described earlier).

Roberts says that had he seen MP two months before, he would have turned her away as untreatable. But having heard of nanobiotics, he put her on them. Two months into treatment MP's chest pains improved, a detectable pulse on the top of the foot developed, and Roberts began EECP. After four months MP's chest pain went away. The left foot pulse was now full, and MP's blood flow to the lower extremities improved. Roberts was also able to discontinue a kidney drug because her kidney function had improved.[9]

Patient BD: improvement despite high CT scores

BD doesn't smoke, his lipids and blood sugar are under control, and he exercises, but the level of his lipoprotein(a)—"really bad" cholesterol—is in the worst 5 percent of the population. This type of cholesterol is designed by nature to be a repair particle. Unfortunately, it also tries to "repair" vessels that have had surgery, thereby blocking them.

In 1991 BD had a heart attack. Angiography demonstrated narrowing of the arteries, so grafts were placed in them. BD returned six months later with a second heart attack, due to closure of one graft. In 1994 another graft closed, so angioplasty was performed. Chest pain recurred in late 1999 because the artery that had undergone angioplasty had renarrowed. BD was left with only one open artery. EECP was carried out and worked well, but chest pain returned in 2001.

BD lived out of town, so travel was an issue. EECP and other therapies require daily visits to a doctor's office. Since nanobiotic therapy does not, it could be done at home.

BD tolerated the nanobiotic well, but his CT score rose after four months. He was disappointed, but agreed to two more months of treatment. His score then fell but was still above where it had been at the start.

At first this might suggest that the nanobiotic didn't work. Yet BD's chest pain had fully resolved for the first time in years. His "good" cho-lesterol (HDL) level rose ten points, and his "really bad" cholesterol level dropped by eleven. His ability to exercise increased measurably, as did other clinical factors. So from a perspective that excluded calcium scores, nanobiotics were working.

Why was there such a mismatch between the CT score and the clinical, laboratory, and stress test findings? It is worth exploring because Roberts often saw this when treating patients with long-standing atherosclerosis and bypass grafts. Here are some of the reasons that he suggests:

In these long-standing coronary disease patients with dense calcification, it may be difficult for the radiologist to determine where calcification ends in [one part of the heart] and where it begins in [another]. The radiologist who reads your first scan may not be the radiologist who reads your second, and the cut-off point is a little subjective, and this can lead to "shifts" in the calcium scores from one vessel to another.

Sometimes, but not always, a metal clip is used to affix the bypass graft to the bypassed artery; this will show up on an Ultrafast CT scan as calcium, the same situation as with the coronary stent—this confuses the reading.[10]

Then there is what Roberts describes as the "blind alley" effect in patients who've had grafts:

The artery is open only over its initial one third, and thus it receives little flow. The artery is occluded in more than one location; portions may be "isolated."

If our goal is only to decalcify the coronary artery and make the CT scan look better, then we have a problem, as we aren't going to be able to get much nanobiotic into these blind alley regions which typically contain the heaviest calcification. We may not, at least not within four months, significantly alter the natural history of calcification progression in [these] regions.

We get plenty of treatment into [other] vessels and into the microcirculation, but these regions don't contain much calcium, so calcium score wise, we have little to show for our work and the patient's efforts.

We are certainly getting nanobiotics into the bypass grafts, but the CT scanners available today aren't able to calcium score the bypass grafts, so any improvement in graft wall calcium goes "unrecognized."

Thus when we treat postbypass patients with nanobiotics their symptoms decrease, their lab values improve, and their stress parameters increase, but the calcium scores over their bypassed vessels may not change—they may even go up, even though the patient is getting better.

For these reasons, I am now typically not obtaining CT scans on my postbypass patients. They have coronary atherosclerosis, so I know that they have a vascular wall nanobacterial infection, and a follow-up scan is often misleading, so why not save the patient some money, and treat them based on symptoms, stress test, and laboratory parameters, which do seem to reflect what [is] actually going on in the patient?[11]

In a later case history of another patient, Roberts adds this important finding about the usefulness of tests for diagnosing progress:

We know that CRP (C-Reactive Protein), the best marker of vascular wall inflammation, is also our best predictor of who will and who will not develop coronary disease, and who will have an adverse coronary event, or experience a complication or recurrence of disease following angioplasty, stent placement, or bypass surgery. Statin cholesterol lowering drugs, antioxidants, and fish oil all have been shown to lower CRP a little, but not like this. We typically see a pronounced drop in CRP when we treat cardiovascular patients with [the nanobiotic], and it may just be that vascular wall inflammation, due to *Nanobacterium sanguineum*, is the culprit underlying this ominous inflammatory marker.[12]

Patient MJ: the case of the "Up-Down Phenomenon"

Among the results identified by Roberts and others is an apparent *increase* in calcium and antibody test scores in the early stages of nanobacteria treatment, followed by a decrease later. There is some difference of opinion among physicians who prescribe nanobiotics as to whether and how much calcium scores go up when patients are initially treated. Some argue that the rise in the score can be attributed to inaccuracies in older technologies that were first used to score patients. Roberts acknowledges this but still maintains that he and other physicians have noticed increases in calcium scores in some patients. He says that one explanation for the increase is that nanobacteria may be able to temporarily evade the treatment and in that interval recalcify. But he emphasizes this is a guess.

The outcome of the discussion will be significant for understanding how calcium scoring and the decalcification process work. Regardless of that, there is agreement that at least antibody scores seem to show a temporary increase. Furthermore, these physicians agree that short-term calcium scoring may be less important to patients' well-being than reductions in other measurable heart disease symptoms that are reliably determined with blood work:

> MJ's four month score increase [after a four-month course of nanobiotics] from 1347 to 3070 is way beyond the natural history of coronary artery calcification (20–80% progression per year, depending on the study), so it must be a treatment related effect. The score got worse, but MJ got better—how can we explain this?[13]

With ongoing therapy, MJ's score fell steadily, until after fourteen months it was at 1209, and according to Roberts, clinically he was "doing great."[14] Roberts qualifies his next observations by stating that they are based on his experience treating patients, his understanding of the scientific literature, and conversations with Gary Mezo and Neva Çiftçioğlu. He emphasizes that he can't back up everything that he says here with a scientific study.

MJ's case . . . serves as the most extreme example to date of the Up-Down Effect . . . How, at least in theory, could we make the patients worse with [nanobiotics]? How could we aggravate their vascular wall Nanobacterial infection?

. . . When we dissolve [nanobacteria's] calcific shelters with EDTA and "unroof" them, the Nanobacteria feel threatened. They respond by . . . [increasing] their growth rate and elaborating copious amounts of biofilm. The large volume of biofilm goo which now surrounds the few Nanobacterial cell bodies begins to lightly calcify . . .

If we took a CT scan at this point, we would score calcium over a large area, even though there are relatively few live Nanobacteria present. If we waited for the biofilm to condense into shelters, then the area involved with calcification would condense.

If we kill the now nonsheltered and thus vulnerable Nanobacteria with tetracycline, then new shelters will not form up. The Nanobacteria will be eradicated and the calcium score will drop . . .

. . . Coronary calcification is rarely evenly distributed within your arteries; this means that different arteries were infected at different times and will have different calcium scores when [nanobiotic] therapy is initiated. Thus each artery will demonstrate the Up-Down Phenomenon at different time points. Thus, at 4 months, we may see . . . a gross Up-Down Phenomena, as in patient MJ.

We are winning the battle and the patient is getting better, and with further therapy the patients will further improve and their calcium score will eventually fall, but at half-time, judging by the CT score alone, it looks as if the Nanobacteria have the upper hand—but they don't; this is simply the Up-Down Phenomenon.[15]

The observations of physicians like Roberts were invaluable in establishing the benefits and side effects of nanobiotics. These doctors took a leap with their patients who were "too far gone" for other treatment. In so doing they laid their reputations on the line.

That same motivation to treat "untreatable" patients sparked other, more conservative cardiologists to look at the therapy.

THE CARDIOLOGISTS' CARDIOLOGIST

On the wall of Dr. Benedict Maniscalco's waiting room is a framed certificate identifying him as being voted one of the "Best Doctors in America."

He is the medical establishment—a conservative cardiologist's cardiologist who doesn't take chances with patients without sober consideration.

Maniscalco is well known in Tampa, Florida, where he has treated tens of thousands of cardiac patients. He was instrumental in developing cardiology facilities in the area. In his own words he likes to stick to proven remedies but also keeps "an open mind" to new approaches.[16]

He knows that cardiology is ultimately a losing battle in that the patient always ends up dying of heart disease or resulting complications. Therefore, every cardiologist considers his or her work successful if the relentless progress of heart disease is only slowed, or in special cases arrested.

As a self-confessed skeptic of new heart treatments, Maniscalco explains what inspired him to try nanobiotics with his patients:

> We've known for 200 years that atherosclerotic plaque was an inflammatory process. And we've always thought and been taught that calcium in a plaque was simply the point in the inflammatory reaction in which the calcium deposition occurred. Maybe it was there to strengthen the repair process.
>
> In the past ten to fifteen years there have been many investigations into the lining of the arteries and plaque, and we have investigated a number of infectious agents. Those investigations by a number of major institutions around the world clearly tell us that infectious agents play a significant role and may cause the initial injury that starts the inflammation that leads to the plaque.
>
> We have had large-scale clinical trials in this country in which we've used antibiotics to treat certain organisms that we thought to be the leading pathogen—mainly *Chlamydia pneumoniae*—and the clinical outcomes have not been encouraging because we've not seen a significant difference.
>
> Gary Mezo presented to me his knowledge of *Nanobacterium sanguineum*. Çiftçioğlu and Kajander demonstrated that *Chlamydia* has a cross-reactive antigen with nanobacteria, which was immediately a very enticing thought that, gee, we're detecting what we think is *Chlamydia*, but it may be something else.
>
> Then I read the paper that Dr. Puskás of Hungary had tried to get published unsuccessfully, in which he isolated nanobacteria from atherosclerotic plaque.
>
> So think of my reaction in this way: I've been a cardiologist for almost thirty years and I haven't cured anyone. I have been involved with bringing relief to thousands of patients and providing state-of-the-art cardiology diagnosis and treatment . . . but "cure" is another thing. So [if] there is possibly a way to approach a plaque, break it down, remove the offending pathogen, and eliminate that plaque, then that's an astounding thought.[17]

Until then, the idea that a heart disease trigger might be found, then reversed, had never been confirmed by experience. For cardiologists such as Maniscalco, it meant possible salvation from a distressing occupational hazard: watching patients whom they'd known for years die of an incurable disease.

HOW MUCH STUDY IS NECESSARY?

In the medical and scientific world, clinical trials are essential, while anecdotal results are just that: anecdotal. No regulatory agency accepts anecdotal evidence as proof. They also won't pay much attention to clinical evidence, such as that presented by James Roberts, unless these data are part of a rigorously controlled, independently monitored study. Patients can be raised from the dead and dance a jig on their graves, but this alone is insufficient when it occurs outside the confines of an orthodox, controlled study.

There are good reasons for this skepticism. Treatments that seem to help patients may be influenced by something that a physician has not considered. On top of that, despite the regulation of medicine by many authorities, mistakes are often made and bad practices still abound.[18]

The best way to minimize these and achieve accurate results is to conduct studies under strict supervision, with independent oversight. To guarantee risk-benefit analysis and protect patient rights, guidelines for conducting and interpreting clinical trial studies are agreed with independent agencies such as institutional review boards (IRBs).

Debates continue over how much study is required prior to a new treatment being adopted, especially in the cases of patients who have no other alternative except death. The argument over expensive studies instead of more immediate treatments has grown acute with incurable diseases such as cancer, AIDS, and heart disease, where billions of dollars and countless clinical trials have often made only halting headway.[19]

Regulatory agencies delay bringing drugs to market until they have undergone time-consuming, exhaustive studies. Meanwhile, thousands die. Pressure to accelerate the process increases as wealthy and famous individuals start dying.

The depth of the controversy is profound. In America, the reaction against conventional drugs and their approval procedures has been manifested by patients making more visits annually to complementary and alternative medicine (CAM) experts than to medical doctors.[20] In 1998 the U.S. National Center for Complementary and Alternative Medicine (NCCAM) was started, signifying the new legitimacy of alternative treatments.

Alongside this, declining profits from conventional treatment and insurers' increasing readiness to cover alternatives have led more than a hundred reputable medical centers to start alternative medicine clinics. Some offer therapies that have been verified through few, if any, clinical trials. Yet they are still administered due to what some say have been convincing anecdotal results.[21]

Some of America's most recognized hospitals are administering alternative treatments based on anecdotal instead of clinical trial results. Is this shift happening because hospitals are submitting to the pressure of financial necessity rather than using good medical judgment? Or is it because conventional treatments don't work for many patients? Or is it that anecdotal results are gaining new respectability based on what has been achieved? You'll find each point debated by those who support or condemn the alternative medicine groundswell. For our purposes here, the point is that treatments with minimal clinical trial background are being adopted regularly by qualified professionals in hospitals.

In this context, the argument that nanobiotics are prematurely prescribed because they suffer from insufficient clinical trial evidence is inconsistent with accepted practice in many medical institutions. This is especially noteworthy for nanobiotics because their active ingredients have been used in large quantities for half a century.

Pressure to bring alternatives more quickly to seriously ill patients has led to a kind of schizophrenia in a research community that is torn between safety and demands for results. For example, the highest form of test result verification is seen as the control-group or "double-blind" approach, where one group is given a placebo with no drug while the other is given the real thing, and researchers testing the results do not know which group they are dealing with. The drawback of such an approach is that it is expensive and lengthy, leading to delays for terminally ill and pain-ridden patients. Therefore, studies that do not use blind verification are sometimes being allowed as a first step to broader introduction of a treatment, with the caveat that the treatment is shown to do no harm, or at least does less harm than the disease it is aimed at controlling. On the other hand a contrary trend has emerged that makes studies more arduous. With a "publish or die" syndrome rampant in the academic community, pressure to produce early results is enormous, and many mistakes have been made. Scandals have erupted over the accuracy and safety of studies. Major research institutions lost their federal funding when patients participating in studies fell ill or died unexpectedly.[22]

As evidence of short-cutting and questionable results mounted, regulatory and research agencies started being more strict about what is a "study" and how it is conducted. Such safeguards involve independent verification by an IRB oversight agency.

HOW ONE NANOBIOTIC TRIAL BEGAN

What does this controversy mean for nanobiotics?

To establish legitimacy for the treatment, Gary Mezo approached a high-level group of physicians and clinical trial experts to measure and validate results in a formal IRB clinical study. Thus began a clinical trial supervised by Dr. Maniscalco under rules established by the Western Institutional Review Board (WIRB).[23]

> This was the first study of a nanobacteria treatment to be done under the auspices of an Institutional Review Board. We wrote a protocol specifically to be followed that was submitted to the Western IRB. The purpose of involving such a review agency is first to protect the patient to make sure that safety precautions are taken and that, for example, patients don't accidentally die due to an inadequately supervised protocol. Secondly, the agency insures that studies are done according to pre-established guidelines and ethical considerations.[24]

Because the patient base of the clinical study was relatively small, it's important to understand what such an analysis may or may not prove under the parameters established.

Maniscalco says that when he and Mezo first met, he was intrigued by the pilot study done on a few patients who had calcification. The significance, he says, was this, "If it's true that increasing amounts of calcium mean increasing amounts of plaque, then if it can be reversed, that would be a phenomenal discovery."[25]

Mezo told Maniscalco that this was what had happened in his earlier unregulated pilot study. After Maniscalco investigated the literature on nanobacteria, he agreed to do the clinical trial under the auspices of an IRB.

The main purpose was to analyze and validate the "before and after" clinical symptoms of patients with heart disease who were treated with the nanobiotic. A main detection method was heart scanning that shows the level of calcium in coronary arteries. Maniscalco talked to some of his heart patients who had a lot of calcification in their arteries and enlisted them for the trial.

Tests for nanobacteria antibodies and antigens were performed, along with electrocardiograms, and tests for CRP (C-reactive protein), cholesterol, and other indicators that signify inflammation in heart disease. Then Maniscalco put the patients on the nanobiotic and started monitoring changes.

> The intended end point was to determine whether a four-month treatment with nanobiotics would lead to a drop in the calcium score as recorded in technology called electron beam computed tomography (EBCT) or Helical Ultrasound Tomography (HCT). [Note: Both methods are used for heart scanning.] We screened about 130 patients. We wanted to have a hundred complete. We ended up with 77 patients who completed it.

An outside review committee of cardiologists then was chosen: "It was their job to confirm that data was collected, that it is in fact what I said it is, and that the protocol is followed properly."[26]

RESULTS

Results of the trial have been published in abstract form and, at the time of writing, were in press at a recognized medical journal. Based on those, Maniscalco has made observations in this chapter and more completely in his own words in the afterword.

> I've observed patients that have had clear changes in their calcium scores. That in itself is remarkable.
>
> In four months we've noted patients who have marked variations in their [nanobacterial] antigen and antibody scores. We had patients coming into the study with an antigen of zero and we started treating them. As we break down the calcium, suddenly the antigen level goes shooting up. Then we treat them and a few months later it's down again. That can only mean to me that we're liberating the source of the antigen from a plaque, and subsequently it becomes detectable and we're killing it. And the antigen falls to zero.
>
> Along with that we've noticed that some patients who have limited functional capacity can double or quadruple [theirs]. For instance, one lady on the treadmill could walk maybe six to nine minutes and now she walks 45 minutes to an hour.
>
> We've noticed patients whose symptoms limited their exercise, but now whose symptoms went away. I have a patient who came in with severe leg pains, no pulses in his lower extremities, and we treated him and the pains went away and the pulses came back.
>
> The other thing that's astounding to me, that I've never seen in thirty years, is that pulses are zero then they come back.[27]

This was the same phenomenon noted earlier by Dr. James Roberts. Maniscalco elaborated:

> There was no ill effect on kidney. No ill effect on liver. No ill effect on bone marrow that I could tell by looking at blood work. And there seemed to be pretty much a strong effect on lowering cholesterol, raising HDL ("good" cholesterol) and lowering LDL ("bad" cholesterol) beyond the [effects of] the therapy that patients were already on.
>
> In general I've learned that patients feel more energetic and better after they've been on it for a while. We've seen decreases in calcium scores, which can only mean that we're decreasing plaque. We've seen fluctuations in antigen (and) antibodies which mean that we're liberating the bacteria and killing them. We've seen changes in functional capacity in symptoms that can't be explained in any other way than in the fact that we treated them.

After the study was completed, Maniscalco continued the treatment, especially with some of his patients who hadn't shown as convincing results: "I'm noticing now that even those whose scores didn't change much in four months continue to get better and their scores are falling precipitously after the trial was over."

DURATION AND SIDE EFFECTS

Side effects are discussed further in the next chapter, but Maniscalco says that in the study he observed, "The only major side effect that made us have to withdraw (one) patient was (an) allergic reaction to a component of the treatment."

He has reached his own conclusions about how long the treatment needs to be applied to be effective for seriously ill patients:

> This is not a treatment that takes one month or four months. This is a long-term treatment. Something that hopefully won't be a year or two all the time, but for people with advanced disease it's going to take quite a long time. Because the more plaque you have the longer you've had the disease. We know that it progresses at 40 percent a year, so it's not going to all go away in four months or eight months.[28]

Furthermore, as Dr. James Roberts had also reported, for a few patients it seems that "nothing happened." Why do some show no improvements? Does it just take the treatment more time to work for them?

Still other patients had to drop out of the study due to an oversensitivity to tetracycline. Will there be another solution for them?

Then there is the suppository. "The toughest part of this whole thing is that the compound includes a suppository," says Maniscalco, "and we're not used to using a suppository except with our children. The suppository has some local side effects that are disturbing to patients, but after a two-week period usually things pretty much settle down."

Does Maniscalco think that we might eventually get around the suppository? "When big pharma [the big pharmaceutical companies] has a will, they have a way and there will be a solution to the suppository."[29]

He hastens to add that this treatment is just the first of a new breed of nanobiotics and that approaches that don't use suppositories are already being developed.

A PATIENT WHO PARTICIPATED IN THE TRIAL

The authors interviewed a small number of randomly selected patients who participated in the first clinical trial shortly after it was completed. Here is one patient's story:

In 1989 JK had a three-way bypass and ten years later a quadruple bypass. In his whole life he'd never had high cholesterol or high blood pressure. Just like about a third of heart patients, he had very few of the traditional telling indicators. Yet heart disease killed both his parents and his grandparents.

> Like most people that go through heart treatment, I got a lot of books and read everything I could about [conventionally accepted causes and treatments]. Frankly, none of it made a lot of sense. The typical science for coronary arteries didn't seem to fit me, and I also found many places where people who did fit [the profile] didn't have the disease. It just wasn't consistent in my layman's mind.
>
> I've always been pretty active. I used to be very active in racing cars, and I raced motorcycles when I was a young man. I was an avid golfer.
>
> I got to the point where I couldn't do a lot of those things anymore. I certainly couldn't race cars. I ended up with angina pain after two or three laps in the car. Playing golf I could not walk the course anymore without angina pain, and that's what really finally convinced me to have the second bypass surgery.
>
> About three months after the surgery I was on a treadmill and one of my arteries collapsed while I was on the treadmill. I just didn't have the energy, and the whole lifestyle wasn't as good as it had been.
>
> Dr. Maniscalco came to me and said, "There's this experimental treatment that you might fit."

So JK started the treatment. After Maniscalco gave him literature, he found some more and read about the treatment himself.

> Right off the bat there was no noticeable difference except that the in-
> digestion was a problem. That went away after about three weeks. After
> a couple of months I just . . . felt better. I got back to the point where I
> could walk eighteen holes, no problem. I even played thirty six holes one
> day with no problem. I'm racing the car now. I just got back from three
> weeks on a motorcycle [tour] in the Alps. Not a single problem.

Before the treatment he was taking Toprol and aspirin, and diltiazem
to control blood pressure and chest pain. When he started the treatment,
Maniscalco added Foltx—a folic acid and vitamin B supplement—and
niacin.

Earlier, two years after his bypass surgery, one of his arteries had dete-
riorated to being blocked. At the end of his nanobiotic treatment another
scan revealed that the blockage was zero.

The treatment also had some side effects:

> One of the things that really felt better was arthritis pain. I don't have
> a severe case . . . I have it in my back and my neck, but my back didn't
> hurt anymore. My neck didn't hurt.

> I've had kidney stones in the past. Starting about the fifth month, I passed
> a kidney stone, and about a week later I passed another kidney stone. I
> went to the urologist and had an x-ray done and had four more kidney
> stones. I told my urologist about the treatment and he pooh-poohed it
> as hocus-pocus, but I gave him the Web site and he came back later and
> said it looked interesting.

JK decided to continue with the treatment on a part-time basis and
does it three to four times a week: "I'm not religious about it now. I am
a convert. I believe in the treatment and I'm going to do what my doctor
recommends."[30] He hasn't discussed getting off his other medicines yet,
but he wants to.

Again, it is important to note that JK is one of the patients who participated in the independently monitored clinical study, so his results can
be confirmed with a high level of confidence.

THE CASE OF DR. C.

Just after Maniscalco had made a presentation at a conference of allergists
to explain preliminary results of a nanobiotics trial, he was approached by
retired physician Dr. C. Various physicians have prescribed the nanobiotic
for themselves, but the case of Dr. C. was especially poignant because it
came as an unsolicited response from a physician whom Maniscalco did
not know.

Dr. C. says that his condition is the classic example of the adage "You can pick your friends but not your relatives" because he had a history of heart disease in his family.

His case was in some ways typical. Knowing the history of the affliction in his family, he had been careful about his diet and exercise, hoping to dodge the coronary bullet. Yet one day while he was golfing, he began to feel a pain in his neck. He tried to ignore it, but some weeks later it came back. When he consulted with a cardiologist friend of his, he was immediately scheduled for an emergency angioplasty where a blocked artery was "ballooned" and a stent inserted to let the blood begin flowing. Some time later the neck pain returned and, as is often the case, it was discovered that the stent had blocked, so the artery had to be reopened.

At an earlier meeting of allergists, Dr. C. had heard about the nanobiotic treatment, so he decided to prescribe it for himself. After six months, he says, his calcium score dropped by at least a quarter. He says that it may have been more than that because, as explained earlier, there are still technical problems in ascertaining the level of calcification in a stent when a heart scan has difficulty differentiating between the stent and calcium. Still, the one-quarter reduction was statistically significant. His stent had not reblocked at that point.

Besides the calcium score reduction, a cataract in one of Dr. C.'s eyes disappeared, leading to cancellation of planned surgery to remove it. When his ophthalmologist searched for the cataract and couldn't find it, he allegedly remarked that he'd never seen such a phenomenon.

In an interview with the authors, Dr. C. said that he experienced no side effects from the treatment except having to be "close to a bathroom" in the morning.[31] He added that he would recommend the treatment.

Keep in mind that Dr. C.'s story contains a combination of clinical and anecdotal information and as such is not an observation from a clinical trial researcher.

TREATMENT FOR OSTEOPOROSIS?

It seems odd to think that nanobiotics might help to relieve conditions where calcium is already being removed from our bones, but that's what some researchers say. Let's look at why nanobiotics work against calcium deposits that afflict our organs yet seemingly not against healthy calcium in our bones.

First, the calcium in our bones is usually isolated from the blood by a thin layer of cell tissue known as "epithelium." This suggests that nanobiotics work far more quickly against exposed calcium phosphate crystals in the blood and arteries, whereas they have more trouble getting into bone calcium. Also, the rogue calcium in our blood vessels and other areas may be the first to go because it represents only a tiny fraction—less than 1 percent—of the total calcium that is elsewhere, in our teeth and bones. Finally, tooth and bone calcium seems to be bound in a different matrix than in the apatite that clogs arteries and veins.[32]

Some researchers hypothesize that nanobiotics may do the opposite from attacking our bones: they may *help to eliminate* conditions that cause loss of bone mass.

Nanobacteria suck calcium out of the blood to form their protective shells. This process may interfere with the normal exchange of calcium that occurs regularly between our blood and bones. When nanobiotics eliminate nanobacteria, the infection can't interfere with that calcium exchange anymore.

This may have implications for conditions such as osteoporosis. Drugs such as bisphosphonates that are used to treat osteoporosis have been shown to be effective in eradicating nanobacteria. However, it may be that something else is required along with the bisphosphonates to get at entrenched calcified nanobacteria. Kajander and his team are exploring this.

THE BIG C

What about cancer? As mentioned earlier, nanobacteria seem to have been found in calcified nodes of ovarian cancer patients. The link between calcium phosphate crystals and cancer is definite. They are often found together. Rapid cell division, inflammation, and DNA transfer are each hallmarks of cancer and of calcium phosphate impacts, but this correlation has been frequently overlooked in cancer research. Might eradication of nanobacteria prevent precancerous processes from erupting? It seems a worthwhile question for cancer researchers to investigate.

There is no clinical trial evidence showing that nanobacteria cause cancer or that nanobiotics help to cure it, because no clinical trial has been conducted around such questions. Financial constraints and skepticism have so far prevented this work. Now that the clues are being uncovered, it may be time for research agencies to pay more attention to the issue.

Meanwhile, let's see if nanobiotics are suitable for most of us.

Eleven

Can We All Be Protected?

The race for nanobacteria treatments is on. As we've seen, many combinations seem to work in the lab, but it may take years for these to go through testing and get into the marketplace. Meanwhile, a triad of EDTA, tetracycline, and nutraceuticals is available now.

This early approach seems to work with seriously ill cardiac patients, but the questions are, will it work for everybody, and how easy is it to use?

According to Dr. James Roberts, who has some of the most extensive experience with nanobiotics, there are limitations:

> Despite all the promising early news about this nanobiotic, it should not be considered a panacea. First, it needs to be tested in larger clinical trials of longer duration before I'm confident of its usefulness. Second, "fluffing" the calcified plaque to allow the tetracycline ample penetration could possibly precipitate angina. Such was the case for one of my patients, who had to withdraw from the study.
>
> For now, I would treat those patients with very high calcium scores or those with angina who have a poor quality of life and are running out of options. This is where the real beauty of nanobiotics for antinanobacterial treatment lies—providing one more card for us physicians to play when the stakes are the highest. Otherwise, there's little we can do when someone's vessels are clogged beyond repair.
>
> Perhaps we'll eventually discover new combinations of procedures.[1]

THE GOOD AND THE BAD

According to physicians who have prescribed nanobiotics, both good and bad clinical and anecdotal results have been observed. These do not occur in every patient. Instead, varying results were seen and not everyone had each type of reaction shown in figure 10.

RISKS

As emphasized throughout this book, every patient should consult with a qualified physician prior to any treatment, and that rule also applies to nanobiotics.

The real and perceived risks of using a treatment for nanobacteria vary depending on a patient's condition. For those who are among the tens of millions suffering from life-threatening circulatory disease, "relative risk" takes on a different meaning compared to the risk for a healthy person who is at only the beginning stages of heart disease and is not slowed or crippled by it. Patients who have shown the most dramatic improvements are those who are worst off. There is a historical reason for this. The treatment was first tried on those who had exhausted other available means. Gary Mezo had made the decision to treat the inoperable, the "cardiac cripples" who had no other options. For these severely ill individuals the relative risks of nanobiotic treatment are usually minuscule compared to the risks of dying from heart disease.

Yet for someone who is not showing symptoms of a calcification-related disease, there may be cause for thought because the treatment hasn't been around long enough to show its warts.

Let's look briefly at each of these risks and who says what about them:

Tetracycline. At one time tetracycline was on the front line of the miracle drug revolution because it used to kill a wide spectrum of bacteria. Then resistance set in and effectiveness diminished, so it is not as widely prescribed now. Most individuals have no trouble with the drug aside from mild stomach upset that usually diminishes after a few days. A rare percentage of the population is allergic. Some patients get severe headaches. Sun sensitivity can also occur. Tetracycline is not recommended for use with young children, but with nanobiotics this is not usually a consideration because the treatment is used primarily in adults.

Misdiagnosis of tetracycline allergies. According to Nanobac Life Sciences, and based on some dermatology studies, nanobacteria are also involved in atopic dermatitis, psoriasis, and eczema.[2] When the nanobiotic

The Good:	Clinical observations:		
	Improvements have been recorded in:		
	Ability to exercise		
	Blood pressure		
	Calcium scores		
	Diabetes symptoms		
	"Good" and "bad" cholesterol		
	Inflammation indicators such as C-reactive protein, erythrocyte sedimentation rate, fibrinogen, and white blood cell count		
	Pulse		
	Triglycerides		
	Stress tests		
	Anecdotal observations:		
	Improvements have been noted in:		
	Age (liver) spot reduction		
	Angina symptoms		
	Arthritic conditions (bursitis and tendinitis)		
	Chronic prostatitis or erectile dysfunction		
	Cognitive abilities and/or memory		
	Eyesight		
	General sense of well-being		
	Kidney stones being passed		
	Psoriasis, eczema, lichen planus, or scleroderma		
	Sex drive		
The Bad:	Clinical observations:		
	Abdominal cramping, loose stools, and occasionally wet gas with symptoms usually subsiding with continued treatment after seven to ten days		
	Mild stomach upset and gas caused by tetracycline		
	Rectal irritation from the suppositories in patients with hemorrhoids		
	Anecdotal observations:		
	Difficulty complying with the regimen		
	Rare cases of angina in patients with a history of angina, which usually goes away after one to two months of treatment		

Figure 10: *Clinical and anecdotal observations from administering the first nanobiotic treatment*

treatment is started, persons with those disorders may have a mild "Herx-heimer reaction" that looks and feels like an allergic reaction but is not.[3] This is a temporary increase of inflammatory symptoms of a disease when antibiotics are administered. Tetracycline can also cause gas, constipation, or stomach upset that then subsides. Earlier, patients sometimes reacted to the apple juice used to mask the taste of the nutraceuticals, then blamed that reaction on the antibiotic. Subsequently, however, the powder was put into capsules, so apple juice isn't required anymore.

Suppositories. Americans are not used to putting things in their rectums because this is not a widely used medical application in the United States, except with children and for nausea. Europeans are less queasy about it because their physicians tend to prescribe suppositories more regularly. Not many drugs are administered rectally over four months, so there is some risk that rectal irritation will develop. There is evidence that irritation of the rectum occurs in lab animals.[4] However, this is also where the issue of relative risk versus benefits comes into play. If you're in your sixties and dying of heart disease, you're unlikely to worry much about rectal or hemorrhoid irritation. If you're in your thirties, then it may be something to weigh against risks posed by kidney stones, heart disease, and other ailments. Finally, the whole discussion about suppositories may be moot if someone finds another delivery mechanism that eliminates suppositories from the treatment.

Unroofing. Once the fibrotic and fatty layers and thick calcium deposits are infiltrated, the exposed nanobacteria get nasty by going from a semi-dormant to suddenly active state, causing them to cluster in the blood. That's why it's important to use the right combination of unroofing chemicals with tetracycline. As pockets of nanobacteria are unroofed, antigen levels go up in patients. This indicates that the nanobacteria have been exposed. If patients do not use the tetracycline or nutraceutical supplement, then they may be at risk from clustering of nanobacteria in areas that are constricted by disease. This could trigger further inflammation or clotting. Also, if the treatment is only partially applied, i.e., only some of the ingredients are used, there is a risk of aggravating the infection. The treatment's developers warn that the absence of a crucial ingredient may be a flaw in other regimens that claim to treat nanobacteria. However, so far there has been no clinical trial comparison to verify this.

A related phenomenon brings up questions about conventional treatments of kidney stones: do doctors unwittingly unleash nanobacteria by destroying nanobacterial calcified shelters in the form of kidney stones with ultrasound lithotripsy treatments? When a stone is pulverized, it may release billions of nanobacterial particles into our systems, triggering the type of regrowth of calcified deposits that doctors often see. There is as yet minimal evidence to support such a hypothesis, but the discoverers of nanobacteria say that this merits further investigation.

The unknown. The nanobiotic approach has been prescribed only since the year 2000, so these are early days. Some doctors say that a few of their patients discontinued the treatment due to a limited tolerance for it. Still, according to physicians interviewed for this book, indicators of potentially serious trouble, such as reduced kidney or liver function or increased heart problems, have not yet shown up in tests.[5]

SALVATION FOR THE COUCH POTATO?

If you think that you can pop a nanobiotic and then be a couch potato, eat badly, drink alcohol heavily, and let your body deteriorate, don't look forward to getting bailed out. The treatment is not a panacea, and patients still need to conduct their lives with due attention to their health.

Still, according to their developers, nanobiotics may help to kick-start the body's own abilities to defend itself, thus improving our chances for staying healthy. The effectiveness may also be enhanced by exercise and a nutritional diet.

PREVENTION?

In patients who are asymptomatic—those who show no clinical signs of illnesses that nanobiotics are designed to treat—the value of preventative application is still unproven. It will take years of testing before it is known whether or to what degree the treatment has preventative value.

ANSWERING THE CRITICS

The arguments between critics and proponents over nanobiotics are summarized this way:

NANOBIOTICS ARE AIMED AT SOMETHING THAT DOESN'T EXIST

Defenders of nanobiotics counter this statement by arguing that the existence of something that generates calcification is well established, although its biological classification is yet to be determined. Therefore, whether it is alive by conventional definitions is not the point. Viruses and prions also fall in the gray zone between being "alive" and being chemical soup, but they still cause disease. In the case of nanobacteria, the real issue is that chemicals targeted at these "entities" have been shown to dissolve calcification.

THERE IS NO EVIDENCE THAT NANOBIOTICS WORK

That statement is incorrect as far as evidence outside the body is concerned. Findings that EDTA and tetracycline together eradicate nanobacteria in vitro have been published by numerous researchers. A few years ago it may have been legitimate to claim a lack of clinical data about whether nanobiotics are effective against calcification in the human body, i.e., in vivo. However, with patients who participated in a clinical study showing improved blood work and inflammation indicators, along with later reductions in calcium scores, there are now sufficient early results to contest the "lack of evidence" claim.

NANOBIOTICS DON'T MEET EXPECTATIONS

Disappointment was expressed earlier by some prescribing physicians that their patients did not reach the level of decalcification that was originally claimed to have been found in a pilot study.[6] Some patients show no reduction with the first treatment, while others show a substantial reduction. This finding is important because it points to how the treatment may work. As described earlier, calcification is often the last thing to go. First, the inflammation must be reduced and the fibrotic cap layers have to be infiltrated. This can take time before drugs can get at the calcification. Here are other factors affecting how fast patients improve:

- Once tissue dies due to total blockage of an artery, any treatment will require more time to help microarteries replace blood flow around the damaged area. Sometimes such regeneration may not occur at all.

- Radiologists who do the comparative "before and after" readings on calcium removal rates are still gaining experience in how to determine percentages on heart scan photographs, especially on older machines. Although state-of-the-art machines and software are more accurate and less risky than invasive cardiac catheterization, the system is still being optimized. This has led some critics to say that the recorded reductions in calcium scores are questionable because they fall within the large margin of error that has been established for reading heart scan images. The developers respond that a recently completed study used newer scanners and software that eliminate much of the error found with older machines.

▣ Clinical results show that antigen and antibody scores that measure the body's response to nanobacteria often increase temporarily as the treatment begins. This is because the nanobacteria are being unroofed in massive quantities, and although they are being eliminated then excreted in urine, their presence can persist for some time.

Nanobiotics are expensive

When considering the cost, the first question to ask is, in relation to what? Compare the suggested retail price of a nanobiotic course of treatment—in 2004 this was about \$275 monthly[7] over four to twelve months—to the cost of open-heart surgery, which runs about \$25,000–\$50,000. Then add the pain, trouble, lost workdays, and risks involved with such surgery, plus the cost of the many drugs that heart patients have to take, running into hundreds or thousands of dollars monthly for the rest of their lives. By contrast, if nanobiotics continue to be effective after a four- to eight-month regimen and patients require only sporadic maintenance treatment after that, then it would represent an exponential saving over heart surgery.

It is suspicious that so few companies offer nanobiotics

Some critics have wondered why, if the treatment is so good, it hasn't taken the world by storm. There are a few clearly understandable reasons for this. Various companies and physicians are pursuing their own therapies now that early clinical results from nanobiotics are apparent. However, they still have to acquire the expertise. There have been technical barriers. Many discoveries had to be made and then combined to identify the culprit and treat it. Scanning methods to measure calcification in the body had to be improved. Tests for discerning nanobacteria from other organisms had to be invented. Ways of detecting and qualifying nanobacteria had to be propagated in the medical community. A method of optimizing EDTA delivery to properly metabolize the chemical had to be invented then put into practice. Regulatory barriers to commercialization are still substantial, causing more delays for companies that want to develop them. Moreover, those companies have to license the treatment or get around existing patents.

Nonetheless, other competitors are getting into the field. For example, one clinic is already prescribing tetracycline along with its chelation therapy. Other physicians have tried their own EDTA-antibiotics combinations. Watch for heavy competition and possible litigation.

At least one other product that uses a different approach is in the marketplace but at the time of writing had not been clinically tested for its impacts on nanobacteria. This treatment, known as "transfer factor," has been used for decades to help the immune system recognize various infections and develop antibodies to them. A product that is claimed to include transfer factor specific to nanobacteria came into the market in 2004, but no results have been published. Transfer factor is not claimed to cure a disease but instead only enhances the body's own defenses against it.[8] This new development will be watched with interest by competing companies.

Some naturally produced and synthetic chemicals haven't yet been commercialized for this specific purpose but may soon be. As mentioned earlier, citrate that is produced by the body may work against nanobacteria. Citrate derivatives are used to treat kidney stones. Chelating chemicals also have effects. Bisphosphonates seem to work as substitutes for EDTA and have been used experimentally to treat osteoporosis.[9]

THE ETHICAL IMPERATIVE

It is ironic that while some critics have asked suspiciously why so few companies developed a treatment years after nanobacteria were discovered, those same critics have resisted the idea of testing nanobiotics.

There are many precedents for such institutional schizophrenia. Prominent among them is the sad history of stomach ulcer treatment, referred to earlier, where a treatment for *Helicobacter pylori* was discovered years before the approach was broadly adopted as a cure for stomach ulcers. The depth of resistance to the idea of an infectious cause was symbolized in the near-comical way that medical authorities were prodded into recognizing the treatment. Barry Marshall, codiscoverer of the antibiotic treatment for ulcers, credits stimulation of interest by researchers not to the material that had been published in medical journals, nor to evidence from patients who were improving or from doctors who had treated them, but instead to a 1990 story in the tabloid press that ran years after the discovery. Alongside stories about alien abductions, the article revealed what had become embarrassingly obvious: there was an easy cure for ulcers. According to Marshall, it was only after the story appeared that more researchers began to pay attention.[10] This shows how medical tradition sometimes remains entrenched until the popular press wakes up to an issue and starts to ask awkward questions.

Defenders of medical tradition point out that for every mistake such as the stomach ulcer episode, there are hundreds of examples where the press got it wrong. Here, the medical profession successfully prevented quack remedies and theories from harming patients. Therefore, it is argued that a few slip-ups shouldn't be used to condemn the whole profession.

This is true. However, the ulcer example shows more than a slip-up. Many say that it is symptomatic of a century of unreasonable opposition to evidence that infection triggers chronic diseases.

Other defenders of established medicine claim that skepticism about nanobiotics cannot be compared to skepticism about a treatment for stomach ulcers because heart disease is more complex than the ulcer process. They argue that it is unlikely for well-known drugs to be as effective against heart disease as others were against stomach ulcers. After all, how could these succeed where billions of dollars in research didn't?

Unfortunately, such dismissiveness mirrors the attitude exhibited earlier toward ulcer treatment, where experts—especially surgeons—scoffed at the idea that a complex process such as ulceration could be cured with known drugs.

Dr. Stephen Sinatra, a physician who supports the nanobiotic treatment, draws this comparison with the unnecessary stomach surgery that persisted for years:

> In the same way, interventional cardiologists are going in and cutting the blood vessels around patients' hearts to bypass plaque-filled arteries in what has become an alarmingly common procedure. We may learn that all that's needed for severely calcified arteries is a course of the right antibiotic.[11]

Here are some troubling questions that the medical profession faces: Will entrenched interests be allowed to further delay nanobiotics from being given the benefit of further clinical trials? Will hundreds of thousands of end-stage heart disease patients continue to be sent home to die without being told about an experimental approach that has shown preliminary success?

That ethical predicament now confronts every cardiologist in medicine today.

◎

We've seen that this early form of nanobiotic may not be for everyone, but it is applicable to a large group of heart disease patients who have no other alternatives.

Unfortunately, another barrier confronting every new treatment is the ballooning cost of medical treatment in general. Who is going to foot the bill?

Twelve

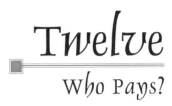

Who Pays?

Treatments for calcific diseases are not just another cost problem; together they are the central problem that sucks up most of our healthcare expenditures.

To compound the strain, after years of medical choices being governed by health maintenance organizations (HMOs) in America and by government programs in other nations, it is clear that Western healthcare systems are in trouble. Exasperated physicians, patients, and insurers agree on one thing: there is a disturbing disconnect between the skyrocketing costs of medical care and the more gradual increases in longevity that we enjoy.

To see how nanobiotics might fit into the cost picture, let's look at what is being tried to control a runaway medical money monster.

Healthcare costs in America testify to what has become a globalized problem. For example, in the year 2000, average cost increases were about four times the inflation rate. Health insurance premiums for employers and employees grew by about 13 percent in 2002, then continued along similar lines in 2003.[1] Such increases were many times the historical percentage improvements in longevity.

And they were not exceptions. They reflected a trend of the past decade. Nor is America alone in this predicament. As insurance premiums for government and private coverage go up in Canada and Europe, the variety of services covered is being reduced.

Some argue that paying on average one-seventh of your income to stay healthy isn't so bad. But the problem is, it doesn't work that way. With obesity and various chronic diseases on the rise, a hot argument has erupted over how healthy these expenditures keep us. Furthermore, with insurers unable or unwilling to keep up with the impacts, the financial burden is falling increasingly on patients when they get sick, instead of being spread out among the population.

Although HMOs, doctors, and drug companies are often blamed, other factors have also been identified:

- The population is getting older, and as it does, health problems and costs increase.

- Western medicine's emphasis on treating instead of preventing disease has proven horrendously expensive as epidemics such as obesity and heart disease grow. Treatments that mask symptoms do not cure disease, so the problems get worse.

- Fraud, government regulation, and pressure by drug and medical equipment company shareholders for profits have worsened the price spiral.

While costs climb, patients don't get the care that they want and doctors can't give the care that they think is required because insurers often won't pay for it and patients can't afford it. Patients and doctors get fed up with being told by third parties what treatments they can get or prescribe.

As a consequence, insurers find themselves being sued for withholding treatments from or dictating them to patients.

THE GRADUAL SHIFT TO PREVENTION

As the patient and physician backlash against cost hikes accelerates, health organizations and governments have begun to cover more preventative healthcare visits.

Alan Iezzi, M.D., F.A.A.F.P., is a practicing physician but also co-founder and medical director of Patient Directed Care, one of a few American companies that broke away from managed care by letting members have unimpeded access to healthcare at a discounted rate, without going through an insurer.[2]

A main focus of the company is prevention because it's cheaper than treatment. Iezzi says that preventative health maintenance makes sense since it reduces disabilities and hospitalizations, while increasing working life via healthy longevity.

Still, he says, one big problem remains: physicians are limited in what they can use for diagnosing or treating diseases because often the preventative tools aren't covered by conventional insurers. For example, with heart disease, Iezzi says that hospitalization and end-stage treatment are the big costs for insurance companies. So why not pay a few hundred dollars for a coronary artery scan as a preventative measure rather than spend a few thousand on catheterization later, when the illness is advanced?[3]

SELF-DIRECTED PLANS

Some employers and insurers are finally beginning to pay for patients to manage their own preventative healthcare via savings and discount systems that minimize red tape.

One concept is based roughly on the U.S. government's Medical Savings Accounts, which give spending discretion to employees. Just like self-directed pension plans, this aims to shift responsibility to workers. The advantage is that it gives the individual more freedom to choose. The tough part is that workers have to be more sophisticated in their approach to healthcare services.

The plans work like this: the employer provides every employee with a tax-free healthcare fund of $1,000–2,000 annually. That doesn't sound like much, but many younger individuals spend less than that annually on healthcare.[4] For older patients, just by coincidence, this is also close to what a course of nanobiotic therapy cost in 2004.

What isn't covered by such medical plans is the cost of catastrophic illness, but there is usually separate lower-cost insurance for such less likely scenarios among the young.

With self-directed plans, employees can use the money for medical services that they want. They can choose their own doctors, get an eye exam, or pay for alternative treatment. In such plans there is no "copay," where an insurer that shares expenses has to approve them; no bureaucrats making medical decisions for patients; and just as importantly, no red tape for getting your money back. If funds are left at year-end, the employee can sometimes, but not always, roll them over into the next year.

The growth in these plans may account for much of the increased research being done by workers themselves on healthcare providers. It may also explain part of the dramatic rise in alternative treatment services—including preventative care—being offered by hospitals across America.[5] The depth of this revolution is only now becoming apparent in the United States, while it has been going on for some time in Europe and Asia.

How many companies are using self-directed plans for their employees? So far a small minority of corporations have offered them, but the schemes seem to be growing in popularity.

Reengineering insurance approvals

A sign of this wave is that some insurers opted to cover the original experimental nanobiotics. Some doctors found the treatment effective and less expensive than traditional therapies. Insurers supported that.

This is the opposite of how things normally happen in insurance. The procedure used to work this way:

It had to be proven beyond a reasonable doubt that something was causing a disease. Then, after exhaustive trials, proof had to be given that symptoms could be treated with a specific regimen. Then and only then, the insurance industry might have looked at it.

That's not the case anymore. Especially for seriously ill patients where conventional approaches have been exhausted, the process is being reengineered because insurers, employers, and patients are looking for cost-effective solutions.

Discounted medical services

The problem with medical savings plans is that they provide limited funds. There is a resulting risk that patients will put off treatment to save money. This is especially true with older patients who may delay treatments that exceed the cost limit of such plans.

For this group, but also for young families who balk at spiraling deductibles in their present insurance, another approach is being tried. A few companies are embarking on what may be the next big approach to healthcare. Dr. Iezzi says that the strategy has been to start with the principle that patients need to direct—and pay directly for—their own care, but not without help. In this case, to provide that help, the insurance company has been cut out of the patient-physician relationship.

"We've eliminated the whole insurance middleman," he says. Patients "can go to anyone who's agreed to provide the discount. They pay directly; there's no claims filing."[6]

A company contracts with healthcare providers to provide discounts to members of the plan. The patient signs up and has access to the network at a prearranged price. The discount is equal to what managed care plans give to physicians right now, but the paperwork has been slashed, so costs are much lower.

Patients are given something like a debit card that lets them pay for services on the spot. The discount runs up to 60–70 percent. According to Iezzi, much of that—up to 30 percent—is generated from less paperwork by cutting out insurance companies.

Due to those reduced costs, most healthcare providers also get paid more than what they'd receive by going through the insurer, so it's attractive to them as well. Moreover, says Iezzi, 90 percent of this type of care is delivered outside hospitals, reducing strain on those systems while saving patients the discomfort of long hospital waiting room visits. Part of that new approach is made possible by the Internet. For example, patients can go to a passworded Web site and get their lab test results quickly.

HOW TO PAY FOR NANOBIOTICS

Since nanobiotics seem to be emerging as a viable option for treating coronary artery disease, Iezzi says that it makes sense to encourage their use. He looks at them from the viewpoint of their potential impacts on healthcare delivery—how the treatment might help to make healthcare more patient directed than the third-party system now in place.

He says that screening for nanobacteria will be offered in the same way. The company hopes to recommend nanobacteria tests to a certain type of patient who might benefit from such a preventative diagnostic tool. That patient would then go to any authorized lab, get the test done, then go to his or her own passworded file on the Web site and see the results. The whole process happens without going to an insurer or hospital.

Will patient-directed discounts work? Several companies are betting on it. Meanwhile, regional offices of a few conventional insurers have already reimbursed patients for experimental nanobiotics.[7] Many of those companies make such payment decisions at the local level on a case-by-case basis. Therefore, just because they pay in one region for one patient does not guarantee that they will pay in every case as a company-wide policy.

Will insurers continue to pay for nanobiotics? That depends on how the treatment develops. As an over-the-counter treatment, it may not be covered, but if combined with an antibiotic prescription, perhaps.

MIGHT NANOBIOTICS PAY FOR THEMSELVES?

Regardless of the outcome, it is safe to say that nanobiotics would be considerably cheaper than open-heart surgery. They may also be viable for older patients because as Medicaid deductibles rise, they find themselves hit with a big monthly bill for heart drugs that they have been told they must take for the rest of their lives. This is inspiring many to look for treatments that deal with the underlying problem instead of just the symptoms. Nanobiotics may be among the few therapies that do this for heart patients. By helping to minimize the need for surgery and other drugs, they may provide a way to cut costs of the coronary drug merry-go-round that many stay stuck on forever.

Nanobiotics might also form part of an affordable preventative strategy that insurers and state agencies can support. Imagine the impacts on healthcare costs if most heart surgeries could be avoided.

So far, the main beneficiaries of nanobiotics have been patients with advanced heart disease. That helps insurers by slashing hospitalization costs. But it also suggests that more research is warranted to determine the effects of nanobiotics on patients with earlier symptoms.

That's where the "who pays?" question also comes in. Research is expensive. Government-sponsored research into nanobacteria and nanobiotics has been painfully slow to get going, while other band-aid treatments receive billions in funding. What is wrong with that picture?

Meanwhile, let's look briefly at where we have been and where we must go to get the nanobacterial monster off our backs for good.

Part III
Steps to Disarming the Trigger

Thirteen

Getting from Here to There

After years of searching, scientists have learned that one of the most widespread medical conditions in existence can be triggered by a previously undetected particle that lurks beneath other diseases. This, along with the knowledge that calcium phosphate deposits cause havoc in the human body, has exposed calcification as an aggressor instead of the innocent bystander that it was once thought to be.

A link has also been discovered between nanobacteria and calcification in the coronary arteries. This turns out to be a new predictor of heart disease.

Researchers have found how to fight the intruder with nanobiotics. Results suggest that when calcification is reduced, the signature inflammation, clotting, and plaque in vascular disease are controlled and reversed. Nanobiotics might therefore work in diseases ranging from kidney stones to cataracts, where calcification is often found.

Other approaches are emerging. The body's own immune response might be enhanced to improve our resistance. We may be able to use certain foods or genetic cues to fight that war. Perhaps the intruder can be eradicated from our food chain. Some nanobacteria sources are known; new nanofiltration techniques might help to make them safer.

THAT WAS THE GOOD NEWS

If patients can be freed of nanobacteria, they still have to be restored to good health and protected from harmful reinfection before anybody can claim they are cured. Until then, it is hard to say if the nanobiotic approach qualifies as a "cure" because it has a therapeutic history of only a few years and has been used primarily with patients who have accumulated heart damage. Therefore, it would be premature to claim that a cure has been found for calcification-related diseases or for calcification alone. However, there have been encouraging results and benefits for patients over earlier treatments. That alone is an achievement.

So many questions are unanswered. How do nanobacteria mineralize? Are there different strains of the pathogen, and does that explain why it flourishes in parts of the body where conditions vary so much? What precise role does it play in heart disease, kidney stones, and other calcification-related conditions?

On the treatment side, does eradicating nanobacteria prevent kidney stone formation? Do the new chemicals that are used to coat arterial stents inadvertently stop nanobacteria from calcifying? Might nanobacteria develop resistance to treatments as other infections have to other drugs? Might nanobiotics be superseded by more effective methods? Why do some patients get better faster than others? Are some of us immune to nanobacteria?

The nanobacterial calcification process remains imprecisely defined, as does its potential role in many diseases. Scientists don't know the final details of nanobacterial nucleic acids, although they have seen glimpses of the genetic building blocks.

Some of the ways that nanobacteria use to enter cells are known, but others are not. It is not known how long they can live, but it seems to be years or perhaps far longer, especially in their dormant state. A few scientists theorize that this form of organism has been around since early life began and that this accounts for the primitive yet effective survival strategy that makes it so hard to find and get rid of.

Other pathogens such as bacteria and viruses, including herpes, *Chlamydia*, and dental germs, have also been found in heart disease. Are they secondary to nanobacteria infections, or do they somehow interact with them at the beginning?

Might nanobacteria cause osteoporosis—loss of bone density—in many women by interfering with the normal calcium exchanges in the body? What role might they play in fetal heart abnormalities associated with calcification? What about the many other diseases that involve calcification?

What about cancer? As described earlier, nanobacteria have been discovered in ovarian cancer. It is known that calcium phosphate crystals found in many cancers are aggressive. They stimulate cell division and provoke the same type of inflammation found near cancers. These crystals in turn have been shown to be generated by nanobacteria. This sequence of nanobacteria-induced crystal generation, inflammation, and rapid cell division is grossly understudied in relation to cancer and warrants far more attention.

To find answers, more work is required with patients where the condition is less advanced. This means working with those in their thirties, forties, and fifties. It also means working with very young patients who have unusual calcific conditions.

Conversely, might some nanobacteria be good for us? There is no evidence of that yet, but if they are so prevalent in our environment, who knows?

The underlying mysteries remain: where did they come from, how old are they, and what form of life are they truly? Were they used by nature millions of years ago to store valuable calcium and phosphate that are essential ingredients for cell life? Are they still used for such a purpose? Are they in our water or vaccines? Are they in food and if yes, how do we get them out?

CLARIFYING THE TERMINOLOGY

Much of the confusion surrounding nanobacteria has come from the name. This might be partially resolved by getting rid of the term "bacteria" in the case of nanoparticles that exhibit nonbacterial properties. The term "nanobes" used by some scientists may warrant investigation as an alternative. However, this is only one of many possibilities. We do not pretend to have answers to the terminology controversy, but we do know that it is time to address it so that instead of mistakenly stuffing these novel particles into traditional boxes scientists can put them into categories that match their properties.

HEALTHY SKEPTICISM OR HEADS IN THE SAND?

Sadly, skepticism about whether nanobacteria exist has delayed investigations, although one would think that such controversy might spur researchers to prove or disprove something instead of discounting it.

With nanobacteria, such a delay might be excused because the discoveries occurred over a range of disciplines that few experts have the background to integrate. The particles were far from being obvious until tools ranging from scanners to specialized antibodies were developed.

At the core, a disturbing undercurrent of disbelief has hampered research, just as with earlier refusals to acknowledge infection in other diseases. Skepticism is not a justification for obstruction. This barrier must be neutralized to get at the truth.

Nanobiotics have also suffered from the same lack of attention that prevented development of antibiotics after their discovery. However, one difference is that antibiotics were newly isolated chemicals whose overall impacts on human health were unknown, whereas the first nanobiotics contain known chemicals that have been in use for decades. Another difference is that many patients are more educated about their medical choices now than when antibiotics were discovered and are more prone to find out for themselves.

Still, the politics of science and medicine being what they are, diligent attention must be paid to verifying the evidence about calcification and how to treat it in a reasonable time frame. The lives of millions of patients may rest on the outcome.

WHAT'S KNOWN AND WHAT'S NEXT

Despite limited resources and support, important discoveries have been made. There are now tests for the particles that trigger inflammation and calcification in the body. There are nanobiotics that according to clinical results reverse markers of atherosclerosis. These are available to millions who might otherwise die or suffer unnecessarily. They may help to relieve the financial and psychological burdens for families and friends.

More study is required. More is under way. But the pace is too slow.

The evidence seems sufficiently compelling to justify a new approach to what may be the most widespread chronic condition on Earth.

Afterword

Miracles happen not in opposition to Nature, but in opposition to what we know of Nature.

—St. Augustine

I n April of 2004, a team led by Dr. Stephen Epstein of the Washington Hospital Center in Washington, D.C., using tests developed by Drs. Olavi Kajander and Neva Çiftçioğlu, succeeded in showing a link between the presence of nanobacteria and high levels of coronary calcification in patients. This was an early step in proving the nanobacteria-atherosclerosis relationship. I was encouraged to see these results because they confirmed my own work in a related area and reaffirmed my reasons for retiring from the practice of invasive cardiology to focus on noninvasive treatment.

I am a reformed invasive cardiologist who used to specialize in surgical procedures for diagnosing and treating diseases of the heart and blood vessels. I founded a major heart institute in Tampa, Florida. After thirty years, when the ravages of wearing a lead apron took their toll, I decided to stop.

In all those years of doing invasive cardiology, I was clearly being a reactive physician. I was reacting to illness in patients who have late-stage cardiovascular disease that is commonly known as "heart disease" or "atherosclerosis." So when I left the laboratory and shredded the lead apron, I decided to take a new look at the primary causes and potential preventions of cardiovascular disease. I got very interested in how atherosclerosis develops. In that process I learned many things more clearly than I had earlier.

The nature of atherosclerosis has eluded us for over two hundred years. We have known for at least that long that it was an inflammatory disease but never understood why and how it begins.

I have been looking at coronary arteries for many years. Like most cardiologists, when I did an angiogram (a photograph of arteries injected with dye), if I saw no narrowing of the outline of the arteries, then I said that the coronary arteries were normal. How wrong my associates and I have been for so long!

In autopsy studies, teenagers and even children ages three and four, who have died of other causes, have been shown to have the early signs of atherosclerosis in the form of fatty streaks. Moreover, a new technology called "intravascular ultrasound" (IVUS) has been used to look at the arteries of donor hearts for transplant patients. This revealed that in those hearts, which we accepted as being free of disease, there was in fact significant disease.

More importantly, we've come to understand that this process is not isolated in the coronary arteries but occurs throughout the arterial system in the body. In the natural course of the development of atherosclerosis there is a deposition of fibrous tissue, cholesterol, cellular components, chemicals, and calcium in the wall of the arteries. What interests me is that the calcium is scattered throughout this collection of cellular material and is in multiple locations. Throughout the body these "deposits" occur or are in various stages of development.

I've been looking at calcium in the coronary arteries all of my professional career and never really understood how it got there. I was taught, as were most cardiologists, that calcium is part of the inflammatory response. Inflammation is the reparative response to an injury in the body's tissues. We were taught that calcium is brought to this location to repair, reinforce, and seal off the area of injury. Yet as we look at that concept, we have to ask ourselves, why in the world would the body deposit calcium, the stuff that bone is made of, in its own arteries? What good would it do?

For the past generation there has been intensive investigation into the process of inflammation and the role that infectious agents might play in the inflammatory process. It is well documented in the laboratory that various viruses and bacteria can produce the inflammatory process leading to atherosclerosis. However, recent antibiotic treatments for such identified pathogens have not shown any effect on the course of the disease. In fact, there has been no statistically significant difference in the outcomes with regard to sudden death or heart attacks. Antibiotic therapy against those pathogens was ineffective.

The questions then become, what could be causing the disease that begins in childhood but does not manifest itself until the fourth, fifth, and sixth decades, and is it associated with both acute and chronic inflammation? Where did the calcium come from, and why does the calcium become more and more dense?

Many of these questions are addressed in this book. Others remain unanswered. We still have a lot to learn, as the authors are correct to point out.

At such an important juncture in medical history I can give one explanation to readers as to why this book is worthwhile:

Recently my colleagues and I completed a clinical trial in which we treated patients with atherosclerosis with a new experimental nanobiotic developed by Gary Mezo and based extensively on discoveries by Dr. Çiftçioğlu and Dr. Kajander about the pathogen *Nanobacterium sanguineum*, or human nanobacterium, and the impacts of certain drugs on it. Based on results that are now being published, the following statements can be made and can be well understood by readers who have read this book:

◙ We can demonstrate reversal of calcium scores.

◙ Indicators of good and bad cholesterol are improving.

◙ Blood serology confirms the presence of the pathogen, while inflammation markers rise and fall as we correspondingly expose and kill it.

◙ We can demonstrate increased functional capacity in patients, along with decreased symptoms.

Whether final outcomes will change is not yet known. Like many preliminary studies, this will require another long-term study identifying all the factors that will allow us to conclude that human nanobacterium is the pathogen that "triggers" the inflammatory process of atherosclerosis and pathologic calcification throughout the body. However, despite controversy over the pathogen's characteristics, it remains my belief that human nanobacterium plays a critical role in cardiovascular disease. Dr. Epstein's work has provided convincing evidence that this is so. So have other findings by Mayo Clinic researchers that clearly indicate the presence of nano-organisms in the aneurysms of heart disease patients.

Finally, the new nanobiotic therapy is effective and perhaps will give us the opportunity to propose a "unifying theory of atherogenesis."

If we think that this is important today, then consider the possibilities for tomorrow. Today there is an epidemic of obesity, not just in the technologically advanced nations, but also in developing countries. This is accelerating the process of atherosclerosis, especially through the development of insulin resistance and diabetes among those who are overweight. If we don't do something about it, then tomorrow this new epidemic will do something horrendous to our record of the past twenty years in which we've reduced the number of fatal heart attacks. Instead, we will see a whole new group of patients who have aggressive and early heart disease.

The cardiovascular monster called "atherosclerosis" is not only ravaging our older population, but it is also gathering force in the dark recesses of our children's arteries. We have much to do in just a few years to protect them. I am certain that this book will help everybody to see that there is more than just hope for a solution.

Most importantly right now, and as is emphasized throughout this book, regardless of how preliminary these discoveries and treatment may be, they provide new hope for critically ill heart patients who have exhausted other conventional means of treatment and who face certain decline to death.

It is fortunate that the discoverers of human nanobacterium chose to look at "what we know of nature" in a different way.

Benedict S. Maniscalco, M.D., F.A.C.C.

Milestones

Here are highlights along the road to discovery of a trigger and treatment for calcification.

The focus here is on *human nanobacteria*, but references to other nano-organisms are included if they have been mentioned in this book. The word "announces," when used below, shows that the date given was the year of publication. If that word is not used, then the date denotes the year when the discovery was reported to have occurred but may not have been published in a journal at that time.

This list was compiled by the authors of this book based on published works and personal interviews.

1985   Olavi Kajander observes nanoscale particles in vitro, forming a community, as contaminants in mammalian cell cultures. He surmises that they may be alive. Labs fail to grow them due to the particles' special properties.

1986   Robert Folk observes nanoscale entities in geological formations, but he does not publish his findings for years.[1]

1986–87   Kajander observes that some of the particles he found seem to have a hard surface.

1987   Kajander discovers the particles in human blood.

1988   Kajander takes the first electron microscope pictures of them and develops polyclonal antibodies to detect them.

1990   Kajander files for a patent for nanobacteria, plus culturing and antibody methods.

1991   Neva Çiftçioğlu and Kajander develop new monoclonal anti-
        bodies to detect nanobacteria.

1992   Kajander is awarded a patent for nanobacteria and related
        detection methods.[2]

1992   Çiftçioğlu discovers that nanobacteria make mineralized "igloo-
        like" structures. These explained the hard surfaces observed
        earlier by Kajander.

1992   Kajander et al. publish one of the first abstracts on blood nano-
        bacteria.[3]

1992   Çiftçioğlu and Kajander optimize the culturing process by
        developing a medium that makes nanobacteria grow quickly
        and produces colonies on solid media.

1993   Kajander and his company optimize methods for detecting
        nanobacteria antigens as a prototype for the commercial meth-
        ods used today.

1996   David McKay et al. announce the discovery of nanoscale organ-
        isms in a meteorite.[4] A controversy over nanobacteria begins.

1997   Çiftçioğlu, Kajander, et al. announce the discovery of potential
        nanobacteria contamination in antibody products.[5]

1997   K. K. Akerman, J. T. Kuikka, Çiftçioğlu, J. Parkkinen, K. A.
        Bergström, I. Kuronen, and Kajander announce the discovery
        that nanobacteria replicate in rabbits, fulfilling part of Koch's
        Postulates.[6]

1998   Çiftçioğlu and Kajander announce discoveries that EDTA
        unroofs nanobacteria and that tetracycline eliminates them,
        then apply for a patent that was later allowed by European and
        American agencies.

1998   Çiftçioğlu and Kajander announce the discovery of nanobacteria
        in kidney stones.[7] The story is covered by journals and news
        services worldwide.

1998   Çiftçioğlu, V. Çiftçioğlu, H. Vali, E. Turcott, and Kajander an-
        nounce the discovery of nanobacteria in dental stones.[8]

1998   Philippa J. R. Uwins et al. announce the discovery of nano-
        organisms ("nanobes") in Australian sandstone. This receives
        media coverage.

1999   László Puskás, who had met Kajander and Çiftçioğlu earlier,
        detects nanobacteria in atherosclerotic plaque and submits his
        findings to journals but cannot get them published in a peer-
        reviewed journal.

1999   Nanobac Oy, a Finnish start-up company, begins using tests for diagnosing nanobacteria in patients with heart and kidney disease.

1999–   Charges against Kajander that his investigations into nano-
2000   bacteria were fraudulent are officially investigated and dismissed as groundless.

1999–   Gary Mezo develops a compounded formula to treat heart
2000   disease. This was later reformulated to include tetracycline, based on Çiftçioğlu's and Kajander's discoveries.

2000   Mezo meets Kajander and Çiftçioğlu, then adds tetracycline to his prescription treatment to neutralize nanobacteria.

2000   Enrique Garcia-Cuerpo et al. fulfill Koch's Postulates for proving nanobacteria as infectious agents.[9]

2000   Thomas Hjelle, Marcia Miller-Hjelle, Çiftçioğlu, et al. announce the discovery of nanobacteria in polycystic kidney disease.[10]

2001   Çiftçioğlu and Kajander announce the detection of nanobacteria in viral vaccines as reported by *Vaccines Today* and *New Scientist*.[11]

2001   First Nanobacteria Symposium held in Kuopio, Finland, brings nanobacteria researchers together.

2002   NanobacLabs (now Nanobac Life Sciences) licenses Nanobac Oy laboratory tests for detecting nanobacteria.

2002   Karl Stetter et al. announce the discovery of *Nanoarchaeum equitans* in volcanic vents and sequence the organism's DNA.

2002   American cardiologists begin to report that their patients have sustained reductions in heart disease markers after treatment with nanobiotics.

2002   Todd Rasmussen et al. duplicate László Puskás's work, finding nanobacteria in atherosclerotic plaque.[12]

2002   Çiftçioğlu and Kajander announce the discovery of contamination of gamma globulin products with nanobacteria.[13]

2002   Benedict Maniscalco et al. conduct the first independently monitored clinical trial of nanobiotics in heart disease patients after being approached by Gary Mezo.

2002   Y. Li, Y. Wen, H. Wei, W. Liu, A. Tan, X. Wu, Q. Wang, and S. Huang of the Second Affiliated Hospital Central South University, Changsha, China, along with Kajander and Çiftçioğlu, announce the discovery of nanobacteria in bile from the gallbladder.[14]

2003   Martin Kerner et al. announce the discovery of nanoscale entities that replicate in bacteria-like ways in polluted river water.[15]

2003   Maniscalco completes the first clinical trial of nanobiotics and announces preliminary significant reductions in calcium scores and other markers of atherosclerosis. Results are published in 2004.[16]

2003   Kajander, Maniscalco, Katja Aho, and Mezo put forward a unified theory of atherogenesis and treatment based on nano-bacteria.[17]

2003   Roland Sedivy and Walter B. Battistutti announce the discovery of nanobacteria in calcified adenocarcinomas in ovarian cancer.[18]

2003   Nanobac Pharmaceuticals Inc. (later Nanobac Life Sciences) becomes the first publicly traded research company to focus exclusively on development of nanobacteria-related products.

2004   Madhu Khullar, S. K. Sharma, S. K. Singh, Pratibha Bajwa, Farooq A. Sheikh, Vandana Relan, and Meera Sharma announce that they have isolated nanobacteria from human renal stones.[19]

2004   The Sino-Finland Nanobacteria Co-Operation Center, an international institute devoted to the study of nanobacteria, is started by the University of Kuopio in Finland and the Second Affiliated Hospital Central South University, Changsha, China.[20]

2004   Tomislav M. Jelic, Amer M. Malas, Samuel S. Groves, Bo Jin, Paul F. Mellen, Garry Osborne, Rod Roque, James G. Rosencrance, and Ho-Huang Chang announce the discovery of nanobacteria in the heart valve of an end-stage diabetes patient.[21]

2004   John Lieske et al. announce that they have found RNA-synthesizing nano-organisms in cardiovascular disease.[22]

2004   Stephen Epstein and Jianhui Zhu discover a correlation between high levels of calcium deposits in coronary arteries of patients and the presence of nanobacteria, using a quick test that can serve as a tool for predicting heart disease.[23]

2004   X. J. Wang, W. Liu , Z. L. Yang, H. Wei, Y. Wen, and Y. G. Li announce preliminary findings of nanobacteria infection levels in healthy subjects in China, concluding that the infection rate of the examined group is approximately 8 percent.[24]

Acknowledgments

T his book would not have been possible without cooperation from Neva Çiftçioğlu, Olavi Kajander, and Gary Mezo, whose insights were invaluable.

Appreciation goes to Alex Edwards, Brady Millican, Bob Parker, John Stanton, Karen Taylor, and the rest of their team for providing valuable updated information.

The authors are indebted to Benedict Maniscalco, who let us witness often-blunt discussions about what has to be done to optimize a treatment for atherosclerosis. Among the physicians who have been prescribing nanobiotics, James C. Roberts gave us keen insights into his experiences, especially with EECP- and EDTA-related therapies. Appreciation goes to Dan Tucker for his insights into immunology. Thanks also to Alan Iezzi for his special insight into the medical insurance industry, Stephen Epstein for observations on nanobacteria tests, and Alan Moore for being the perennial skeptic.

To the critics of nanobacteria who took the time to respond to our questions, their contribution was valuable.

To the medical reviewers who consented to check this text: thank you. We also extend our thanks to Yossef Av-Gay, George Fox, and Karl Stetter for proofing selected segments and to Katja Aho for providing study materials and drawing our attention to the discoveries of nanoparticles in water.

To Steve Mulhall, Patrick Moore, and Rena Subotnik who critiqued our work from different perspectives, it was appreciated.

Thanks go to Lisa Grant and The Writers' Collective, who are pioneering a new way of publishing that gives authors more control over their work; to Fritz Stork for getting things done on time; and to our cover designer, interior designer, and copy editors for their diligent work.

Most of all, thanks to the patients who let us into parts of their lives normally reserved for the physician-patient relationship. We hope that this book justifies the trust that you've put in us so that others may benefit.

Appendices

Plain Language Glossary

This glossary is for nonmedical readers who want to understand the technical terms used in this book. The explanations are not just borrowed from medical dictionaries but instead have been customized to explain how they relate to calcification, nanobacteria, and various diseases. There is, to our knowledge, no other glossary that explains such terms in this context.

Anecdotal evidence—Findings that are based on casual observations or indications rather than rigorous or scientific analysis. "I feel better" and "My pain seemed to go away" are anecdotal statements. Objective clinical evidence does not depend on anecdotal reports. In this book, observations about patients who took treatment for nanobacterial infections are divided into anecdotal and clinical evidence. *See* clinical evidence.

Aneurysm—A dangerous blood-filled dilation of a blood vessel caused by disease or weakening of the vessel's wall. This can cut off blood supply and cause death. Researchers theorize that calcification can provoke aneurysms. Calcified nanobacteria have been found in aneurysms.

Angina—Acute pain and a feeling of tightness brought on by reduced oxygen supply to the heart, often associated with partial blockage of the coronary arteries by calcified deposits.

Angiogram—An x-ray of blood vessels that shows obstructions in the vessels when the patient receives an injection of dye to outline the vessels on the x-ray. This is regarded as being more accurate but more risky than a CT scan and less accurate than catheterization, when an instrument is inserted directly into the vessel. The accuracy of angiograms in showing inflammation and calcification is questionable because inflammation can vary in patients from time to time, and some calcium deposits won't show up on an angiogram. *See also* CT scan.

Angioplasty—Widening of a partially or fully blocked artery by inserting a hollow wire that is then inflated. Angioplasties often reblock over months or years. It is theorized that the procedure may release large amounts of nanobacteria that trigger the reblocking process.

Ankylosing spondylitis—Chronic inflammation of vertebrae in the spine. It can immobilize a patient. Calcification is found here.

Antibodies—Substances that are manufactured by the immune system to deal with infection. Because these tools precisely "recognize" and bind to specific shapes on other molecules, antibody binding is also used by researchers to identify organisms. In the case of nanobacteria, antibodies have been engineered to test for their presence.

Antigens—Substances that cause an immune reaction in the body. A bacteria, virus, or other pathogen can be an antigen. These are also used as markers to identify the presence of infections such as nanobacteria.

Apatite—A form of calcium phosphate mineral found in rocks, bone, teeth, kidney stones, and atherosclerosis. *See* calcium phosphate.

Arteriosclerosis—A vascular disease characterized by thickening and hardening of artery walls.

Atherosclerosis—One of several types of arteriosclerosis. Characterized by the deposition of plaques containing cholesterol and lipids on or in the innermost layer of the walls of large and medium-sized arteries. Calcification and nano-bacteria have been found in atherosclerosis.

Atopic dermatitis—Inflammation of the skin resulting from a hereditary predisposition to developing hypersensitivity reactions. Calcification is in this condition.

Biofilm—A film consisting of organisms or their by-products. It lets the organisms stick to a surface, but can also have many other functions, for example, as a nutrient, defensive mechanism, or disguise. Nanobacteria have been observed to produce biofilm for such purposes.

Bisphosphonates—Drugs used to prevent and treat osteoporosis. Possible alternatives to the use of EDTA in nanobiotic treatments. They have also been shown to eliminate nanobacteria after the protective calcium layer has been removed.

Bromelain—A protein-digesting enzyme, derived from pineapple, that is thought to help fight plaque. It is a natural blood thinner that lessens the risk of blood clots and also reduces inflammation. It is an ingredient of a nutraceutical supplement aimed at removing cardiovascular plaque.

Calcification (pathological)—Deposition of calcium compounds in parts of the body where they are not supposed to be, producing harmful results consistent with the pathogenic behavior of an organism. Terms used by physicians to describe calcification in the body are in figure 2. *See also* calcium phosphate.

Calcium—A basic mineral, part of the periodic table of elements. The most plentiful mineral in the human body, it is essential for life and is found in our bones, teeth, and cells. Calcium combines readily with many other chemicals, which is one reason it is so useful for life processes. It is also a basis for calcification in disease.

Calcium phosphate—A combination of calcium and phosphorus forming a calcium mineral salt that is found in many calcium deposits in the body. It is toxic to cells and human tissue. *See* apatite.

Calcium score—A calculation that shows the buildup of calcium salts in the arteries. This is done, for example, with electron beam computed tomography (EBCT).

Cardiac catheterization—Inserting a tube into an artery to check for blockage.

Cardiomyopathy—A disease of the heart muscle that causes it to lose its pumping strength. Calcification has been associated with this condition.

Chelation therapy—A treatment to remove heavy metals such as lead from the blood. A common form is intravenous chelation, where a solution containing chelating agents is injected into the body along with mineral supplements to balance the effects on the body. The chemical binds with heavy metals. Then the combination is excreted in urine.

Cholesterol:

> **Good HDL, or high-density lipoproteins**—Often referred to as "good cholesterol." HDL carries cholesterol from your tissues and returns it to the liver. It is called "good" because higher levels of HDL allegedly reduce your risk of developing cardiovascular disease.

> **Bad LDL, or low-density lipoproteins**—Carries the cholesterol from the liver to the other tissues. It is called "bad" because higher levels of LDL allegedly increase your risk of developing cardiovascular diseases.

> **Indifferent**—Some physicians argue that cholesterol does not cause heart disease and is not a reliable predictor of who may have a heart attack.[1]

Citrate—Also known as citric acid. A chemical commonly found in fruit and used as a food additive. It binds calcium and may be one of the body's natural ways of fighting nanobacteria. It is also effective against nanobacteria at concentrations that can be reached by oral or intravenous treatments.

Clinical evidence—Something that is based on direct observation of a patient by a qualified physician. Clinical diagnosis, study, trial, and proof are each predicated on such observations. For example, clinical evidence of changes in a heart patient's condition includes measurements of blood pressure, stress, pulse, "good" and "bad" cholesterol, triglycerides, calcification, inflammation indicators such as C-reactive protein, erythrocyte sedimentation rate, fibrinogen, and leukocyte (white blood cell) count. These are fundamental to understanding whether a treatment aimed at nanobacterial infection also has impacts on heart disease. They are also different from anecdotal evidence, which is far less measurable.

CoQ$_{10}$—A naturally occurring nutrient that helps each cell of the body to produce energy. It is a popular supplement used to fight heart disease. It is claimed to lower the incidence of angina attacks, arrhythmias, cardiomyopathy, congestive heart failure, heart valve irregularities, hypertension, mitral valve prolapse, and periodontal disease. It is an ingredient of a nutraceutical supplement aimed at removing cardiovascular plaque.

CRP, C-reactive protein—An indicator of inflammation that is used to predict heart attack risk in healthy adults. Since the role of inflammation in heart disease is crucial, the role of CRP is becoming increasingly important as a measure of that inflammation. Although CRP is a good predictor, it is not yet known if lowering CRP levels alone reduces the risk of cardiovascular disease.[2]

CT scan, cardiac tomography—A form of x-ray used to provide cross-sectional images of the chest, including the heart and great vessels. It can be used to show calcification but is considered an older technology. For newer technology, *see* electron beam computed tomography.

Diabetes—A disorder characterized by excessive urination and thirst. It is often associated with heart disease. Overweight individuals are subject to becoming diabetic. Calcification is often associated with advanced diabetes.

DNA, deoxyribonucleic acid—Considered one of the building blocks of life and a basis for genetic science. A nucleic acid carries the genetic information in the cell. Some scientists claim that they have found the building blocks for DNA in nanobacteria.

EDTA, ethylenediaminetetraacetic acid—A broadly used government-approved food preservative and the preferred treatment for lead poisoning. Once in the blood it binds to heavy metals and the resulting combination of EDTA, metals, and minerals is excreted during urination. EDTA is a central ingredient of a nutraceutical supplement aimed at removing cardiovascular plaque. *See* chelation therapy.

EECP, enhanced external counter pulsation—A procedure where pneumatic cuffs are placed over the patient's lower extremities, then inflated and deflated repeatedly. This drives oxygenated blood backward from the lower parts of the body into the heart. This pressure stimulates formation of small natural "bypasses."

Electron beam computed tomography, EBCT—A fast form of x-ray imaging technology, also known as an "ultrafast CT scan" or a "rapid CT scan." An EBCT scan takes about ninety seconds and detects calcium deposits associated with heart disease and other ailments.[3] It can take multiple images of the heart within the time of a single heartbeat, providing details about the heart's function and structures and slashing the time required for a clinical study.

Endotoxin—A toxin produced by bacteria and by nanobacteria that harms other cells and often elicits an immune reaction by the body.

Enzymes—Chemical compounds that help a cell to speed up reactions. Many enzymes are ingredients in a nutraceutical supplement aimed at removing cardiovascular plaque.

Epithelium—A thin layer of cells that covers the internal and external surfaces of the body, including body cavities, ducts, and vessels.

Fetal bovine serum, FBS—An extract from baby cow blood used to grow cells for experiments and develop vaccines. The serum has been found to be contaminated with nanobacteria.

Fibrinogen—A protein in blood plasma that is essential for the coagulation or thickening of blood. It is one of the indicators of heart disease. It is used by the body to close off injured blood vessel walls. Elevated levels suggest that the atherosclerotic process is occurring.[4]

Grapeseed extract—An antioxidant used to maintain the health of small blood vessels. It is an ingredient of a nutraceutical supplement aimed at removing cardiovascular plaque.

Hawthorn berry—A herb claimed to lower cholesterol, normalize blood pressure, and reduce inflammation. It is an ingredient of a nutraceutical supplement aimed at removing cardiovascular plaque.

HDL—*See* cholesterol.

Herxheimer reaction—Nicknamed "herx" after Jarisch-Herxheimer, it is a temporary increase of symptoms of a disease when some drugs are administered. It can seem like an allergic reaction to an antibiotic, but it is not.

High blood pressure, hypertension—Blood pressure is the force of blood against the walls of arteries. It rises and falls during the day. When it stays elevated over time, it is called high blood pressure or hypertension. This is considered a measure of stroke or heart attack risk.[5]

In vitro—An artificial environment outside the body, such as a test tube or petri dish. Many biological experiments, such as culturing of bacteria and nanobacteria, are done in vitro, as opposed to in vivo (inside the body). This is done to ease observation and manipulation but also eliminates risk to patients.

In vivo—The environment in the body, as opposed to in vitro per above.

Inflammation—A normally healthy immune system response resulting from injury to tissue. It is characterized by swelling of the surrounding area when capillaries make themselves more permeable to let antibodies and repair cells reach the site of injury to get rid of pathogens and start the healing process. Discoverers of nanobacteria theorize that injuries caused by nanobacteria lead to a persistent inflammatory response, which is not healthy.

Intravascular ultrasound, IVUS—An imaging procedure used to show blockage in coronary arteries. This is regarded as being more accurate than some other procedures because an ultrasound device is inserted directly into the artery instead of the image being taken only from outside the body.

L-arginine—An amino acid that helps blood vessels stay flexible to improve circulation. It also helps the body to fix damaged tissue and bone. It is an ingredient of a nutraceutical supplement aimed at removing cardiovascular plaque.

L-lysine—An essential amino acid that cannot be manufactured by the human body. The only source of L-lysine is foods, such as vegetables and grains, or supplements. It promotes absorption of calcium and production of enzymes. It is an ingredient of a nutraceutical supplement aimed at removing cardiovascular plaque.

L-ornithine—An amino acid that stimulates the release of growth hormone from the pituitary gland for wound healing. It is used as a dietary supplement. It is an ingredient of a nutraceutical supplement aimed at removing cardiovascular plaque.

LDL—*See* cholesterol.

Lipid—A type of fat that includes some natural oils or waxes. It stores energy and carries vitamins.[6] It is among the basic components of a cell that helps give cells structure. Cholesterol and triglycerides are lipids. In heart disease lipids build up in the soft plaque that gums up blood vessels.

Macular degeneration—A condition in which cells in a specific part of the eye degenerate, resulting in blurred vision and ultimately blindness. Calcification has been found in this disease.

MRI, magnetic resonance imaging—A noninvasive procedure that uses powerful magnets and radio waves to construct pictures of the body. This is part of a group of technologies that show obstructions such as calcification and cancers. An MRA, or magnetic resonance angiogram, is a special type of imaging that creates three-dimensional reconstructions of vessels containing flowing blood and is often used when conventional angiography cannot be performed.[7]

Mycoplasma—A sometimes toxic microorganism that lacks a cell wall and that is so small it often gets through filters and contaminates the serum in which biological experiments are done. One species causes a type of pneumonia in humans.

Nanobacteria (human)—A tentative name given to nanometer-scale entities that self-replicate in the body and manufacture carbonate apatite structures (calcium phosphate mineral). *See* "An important note on definitions" at the beginning of this book for a list of the various terms used to describe nanobacteria.

Nanobiotics—Chemicals that eradicate nanobacteria. However, the term is also used to describe other medical applications that operate at the scale of billions of a meter.

Nanometer—One billionth of a meter.

Nano-organism—There is no official definition for this term, but it is used in this book to describe self-replicating nanoparticles that usually measure less than one millionth of a meter in diameter.

Niacin (vitamin B$_3$)—A vitamin used in many ways by the body. In relation to heart disease, it is found to lower lipoprotein(a) (a form of cholesterol) and widen blood vessels. Found naturally in meat, poultry, fish, and vegetables, it is also an ingredient of a nutraceutical supplement aimed at removing cardiovascular plaque.

Nucleic acid—A chemical building block of life. It can be either DNA or RNA. So far, nucleic acid has been found in all living things. *See* DNA, RNA.

Papain—An enzyme used as a digestive aid. It is derived from papaya and certain other plants. It is used in commercial applications such as meat tenderizers. It is also used to treat edemas, to treat inflammatory processes, and in the acceleration of wound healing. It is an ingredient of a nutraceutical supplement aimed at removing cardiovascular plaque.

PATCH study—PATCH stands for Program to Assess Alternative Treatment Strategies to Achieve Cardiac Health.[8] This name was applied to a controversial study done to evaluate the impacts of EDTA intravenous chelation on cardiovascular disease. Results of the study suggested no benefits arising from chelation, but the methodology has been criticized by chelation proponents. This controversy may be settled by a study being done by the National Institutes of Health.

Pathogen—An agent—usually a microorganism—that causes disease. Nanobacteria are considered to be pathogens.

Phosphorus—After calcium the most abundant element in the human body mainly in the form of phosphate in the bones and teeth. Like calcium, phosphorus is essential for many cell functions. But it is also part of calcium phosphate deposits that make up harmful calcification.

Prion—An infectious particle in mad cow disease and Creutzfeldt-Jakob disease in humans. It does not produce DNA or RNA and is not considered to be alive but is dangerous nonetheless. It is the smallest known infectious particle.

Psoriasis—A noncontagious inflammatory skin disease characterized by recurring reddish patches covered with silvery scales. These scales contain calcium deposits.

Rapid CT scan—*See* electron beam computed tomography.

Renal disease—Illness associated with the kidneys and often with calcification.

Restenosis—Renarrowing or closing of a blood vessel that has already been opened surgically, e.g., by angioplasty.

RNA, Ribonucleic acid—A transmitter of genetic information in every cell. It is essential for cell replication. Some scientists say they have found RNA in nanobacteria.

Scleroderma—A pathological thickening and hardening of the skin associated with calcification.

Sedimentation rate or erythrocyte sedimentation rate, ESR—A test that measures the distance that red blood cells settle in unclotted blood toward the bottom of a specially marked test tube in one hour. This is used to monitor inflammatory disease. It is one measure of rheumatoid arthritis, heart, and kidney disease.[9]

Selenium—An essential trace element in the body that we get when we eat foods that take it up from the soil. It is said to prevent very rapid heartbeat, lower high concentrations of cholesterol or triglycerides, and improve diabetic symptoms, congestive heart failure, and cardiomyopathy. It is an ingredient of a nutraceutical supplement aimed at removing cardiovascular plaque.

Statins—A group of drugs used to lower bad cholesterol levels by inhibiting a key enzyme involved in the biosynthesis of cholesterol. Statins have also been discovered to slow the progression of calcification in arteries, but the key word here is "slow," rather than reverse. Statins have not been found to reverse the existing buildup of calcified deposits.[10]

Stent—A tube inserted into a blood vessel to restore blood flow when buildups block it. Stents often get blocked, and it has been theorized that nanobacteria contribute to this blockage. Some newer stents are coated with drugs to try to prevent blockage.

Stress test—Also known as an exercise electrocardiogram, this test measures the heart's response to an increased demand for oxygen brought on by exercise. It is used as a measure of cardiovascular disease.

Tetracycline—Tetracycline hydrochloride, a broad-spectrum antibiotic used to fight bacterial infections. It is a yellow crystalline compound that is synthesized or derived from microorganisms known as "streptomyces." Researchers have found that tetracycline neutralizes unencased nanobacteria and may also have other beneficial impacts on infection in heart disease.

Thrombosis—The obstruction of a blood vessel by a clot. Clotting is a healthy reaction of the body to injury, but it gets out of hand when it occurs in blocked blood vessels and often leads to death. Nanobacteria may spark clotting in arteries because they bind a substance known as "prothrombin."

Transfer factors, TFs—Protein molecules produced by immune cells that let the immune system "remember" conditions for which immunity has already been established. TFs help to alert immune cells to impending danger. They can be transferred from one cell to another, hence the name "transfer factor." It is claimed that some transfer factors recognize nanobacteria and help the body to fight them.

Triglyceride—A type of fat produced by the body to store energy. It is measured as a mild risk factor for coronary artery disease. *See also* lipid.

Trypsin—An enzyme that helps digestion in the small intestine. It also combats inflammation. It is an ingredient of a nutraceutical supplement aimed at removing cardiovascular plaque.

Ultrafast or rapid CT scan—*See* electron beam computed tomography.

Vascular disease—Blockage of blood vessels due to swelling, plaque, and hard deposits.

Vascular system—A network of vessels that carry blood or lymph through the body.

White blood cell count—A high white blood cell count indicates infection or inflammation that has activated the body's immune response. When taken with other test results, such as triglycerides and C-reactive protein, it can indicate inflammation in heart disease.

Who's Who in the World of Calcification and Nanobacteria

Hundreds of researchers, physicians, and other experts are now involved with nanobacteria or measuring their impacts. This list shows some of the major participants and their roles but is not exhaustive. It focuses on human nanobacteria rather than the much larger world of nanobacteria outside the human body, although some players in the wider field are named.

RESEARCHERS

Katja M. Aho, M.Sc., University of Kuopio, Department of Biochemistry, Kuopio, Finland: Collaborates with Olavi Kajander on researching and describing the challenges associated with characterizing nanobacteria.

Kari K. Akerman, University of Kuopio, A. I. Virtanen Institute, Department of Biochemistry and Biotechnology, Kuopio, Finland: Collaborated with Olavi Kajander on scanning electron microscopy in relation to nanobacteria.

Yossef Av-Gay, Ph.D., Division of Infectious Diseases, University of British Columbia and Vancouver Hospital and Health Sciences Centre, Vancouver, Canada: Works on characterizing human naobacteria.

Dennis A. Carson, M.D., Ph.D., University of California at San Diego, former dean, Faculty of Medicine; Director, the Sam and Rose Stein Institute for Research on Aging, La Jolla, California, United States, member, National Academy of Sciences:Postulated that most extraskeletal calcification may be caused by nanobacteria.

David Y. Chan, M.D., Johns Hopkins Hospital, James Buchanan Brady Urological Institute, Baltimore, Maryland, United States: Urologist who did research on nanobacteria and formation of kidney stones.

Neva Çiftçioğlu, Ph.D., Universities Space Research Association, Division of Space Life Sciences, Houston, Texas, United States: Cofounded Nanobac Oy, Finland. Plays a leading role in human nanobacteria research with Olavi Kajander. Codiscovered methods for culturing and detecting nanobacteria. Accelerated discoveries by reducing the time it took to culture nanobacteria and by developing antibody methods to detect them in mammals such as humans. Did pioneering research on human nanobacteria relating to space exploration while working at Johnson Space Center, NASA.

Vefa Çiftçioğlu, D.D.S., Ankara, Turkey: Copublished a paper with his sister Neva Çiftçioğlu on nanobacteria and dental stones.

Franklin Cockerill, Ph.D., M.D., Mayo Clinic, Chief of Microbiology, Infectious Diseases, Rochester, Minnesota, United States: Known for his work on the anthrax vaccine. Heads a research team working on the basic science of nanobacteria diagnostics and plans to sequence the genome of nanobacteria.

Fredric Coe, M.D., Professor, University of Chicago, Illinois, United States: A leading urology researcher in elimination of kidney stones. Currently examining the cause of calcification in kidney disease.

Stephen E. Epstein, M.D., Director, Cardiovascular Research Institute, Washington Hospital Center, Washington D.C., United States; former head of the National Heart, Lung and Blood Institute (NHLBI): Along with his associate Dr. Jianhui Zhu, conducted a groundbreaking study that identified a link between the presence of nanobacteria and the level of coronary artery calcification in heart patients.

Paul W. Ewald, Ph.D., Amherst College, Amherst, New York, United States: Leading investigator into infection as a cause of heart and other diseases. Has published several books on the topic. Has spoken briefly on the potential role of nanobacteria in atherosclerosis.

Enrique Garcia-Cuerpo, M.D., Alcala University, Department of Medicine, Madrid, Spain: Copublished work on kidney stones and nanobacteria, especially showing how nanobacteria cause disease. Has written a book about his findings.

Rauno Harvima, M.D., Kuopio University Hospital, Department of Dermatology, Kuopio, Finland: Researches the relationship between dermatological calcification and nanobacteria in psoriasis, eczema, lichen planus, atopic dermatitis, and scleroderma.

J. Thomas Hjelle, Ph.D., University of Illinois College of Medicine at Peoria, Departments of Biomedical and Therapeutic Sciences, Peoria, Illinois, United States: Researches the role nanobacteria may play in polycystic kidney disease and kidney stones, pineal calcification, and brain sand.

Martin Holmberg, M.D., Uppsala University, Department of Medical Sciences, Uppsala, Sweden: Swedish scientist working on nanobacteria detection in serum.

Tomislav M. Jelic, M.D., Ph.D., Department of Pathology, Memorial Hospital, Charleston Area Medical Center, Charleston, West Virginia, United States: Co-published the discovery of nanobacteria-caused mitral valve calciphylaxis in a man with diabetic renal failure. Coresearchers are Amer M. Malas, Samuel S. Groves, Bo Jin, Paul F. Mellen, Garry Osborne, Rod Roque, James G. Rosencrance, and Ho-Huang Chang.

E. Olavi Kajander, M.D., Ph.D., Nanobac Oy, Kuopio, Finland; Nanobac Life Sciences, Tampa, Florida, United States: The leading researcher in development of nanobiotic treatments and with Neva Çiftçioğlu in nanobacteria diagnostics. Discovered and patented *Nanobacterium sanguineum*. Codevised ways of culturing and testing for it. Codeveloped and patented the first method for eliminating the pathogen. Codeveloped nanobacteria tests.

Madhu Khullar, M.D., Additional Professor, Department of Experiment Medicine and Biotechnology, Postgraduate Institute of Medical Education and Research, Chandigarh, India: Copublished research on lifelike characteristics of nanobacteria from human renal stones. Coresearchers are S. K. Sharma, S. K. Singh, P. Bajwa, F. A. Sheikh, V. Relan, and M. Sharma.

Ilpo Kuronen, University of Kuopio, A. I. Virtanen Institute, Department of Clinical Chemistry, Kuopio, Finland: Coresearcher on nanobacteria.

Hilary M. Lapin-Scott, Ph.D., Professor, Exeter University, Biological Sciences, Exeter, United Kingdom: Along with her colleague S. Burton, researched culturability and biofilm formation related to nanobacteria.

Li Yong Guo, Professor of Surgery, Vice President, The Second Xiang Ya Hospital of Central South University, Changsha, Hunan, P.R. China: Copublished research on nanobacteria in serum, bile, and gallbladder mucosa of cholecystolithiasis patients. Heads the nanobacteria research team of the Sino-Finland Nanobacteria Co-Operation Center at the Second Affiliated Hospital Central South University. Coresearchers are Y. Wen, Z. L. Yang, X. J. Wang, H. Wei, W. Liu, A. L. Tan, X. Y. Miao, Q. W. Wang, S. F. Huang, E. O. Kajander, and N. Çiftçioğlu.

John C. Lieske, M.D., Mayo Medical School, Assistant Professor of Medicine, Research Chair Division of Nephrology, Rochester, Minnesota, United States: Works with multidisciplinary group at Mayo to study the pathogenic role of nanobacteria in human disease, especially kidney stones, polycystic kidney disease, and atherosclerosis.

Gary S. Mezo, A.R.N.P., P.A., Founder, NanobacLabs, Tampa, Florida, United States: Developed the prescription nanobiotic NanobacTX, the first treatment deliberately aimed at eliminating nanobacteria in the human body. Codeveloped the NanobacTEST U/A with Dr. Kajander. Initiated the first independently verified clinical studies on the medical impacts of a nanobiotic.

Alan Miller, M.D., Professor of Medicine, University of Florida Health Science Center, Division of Cardiology, Jacksonville, Florida, United States: Served on the cardiology review board for the first clinical study of the effects of the nanobiotic NanobacTX in heart patients (NanobacTX-ACES II Cardiology Study).

Virginia M. Miller, Ph.D., Professor of Surgery, Professor of Physiology, Mayo Medical School, Rochester, Minnesota, United States: Researches the relationship between arteriosclerosis and nanobacteria. Copublished studies on detection of nanobacteria in aneurysms.

Marcia Miller-Hjelle, Ph.D., A.B.M.M., University of Illinois College of Medicine at Peoria, Departments of Biomedical and Therapeutic Sciences, Peoria, Illinois, United States: Researches the role nanobacteria may play in polycystic kidney disease and kidney stones, pineal calcification, and brain sand.

László Puskás, Ph.D., Hungarian Academy of Sciences, DNA-Chip Laboratory, Biological Research Center, Szeged, Hungary: Discovered nanobacteria in arteriosclerotic plaque.

Todd E. Rasmussen, M.D., Mayo Clinic and Foundation, Rochester, Minnesota, United States: Coresearches nanobacteria in arteriosclerotic plaque with the Austin Heart Center at the University of Texas.

George P. Rodgers, M.D., F.A.C.C., University of Texas, Austin Heart Center, Austin, Texas, United States: Coresearches nanobacteria in arteriosclerotic plaque with the Mayo Clinic.

Roland Sedivy, Professor of Pathology, Department of Clinical Pathology, University Hospital Vienna, Vienna, Austria: Copublished with W. B. Battistutti research on the detection of nanobacteria in ovarian cancer.

Vardit Segal, Technion-Israel Institute of Technology, Leonard and Diane Sherman Center for Research in Biomaterials, Department of Biomedical Engineering, Haifa, Israel: Copublished with Olavi Kajander about nanobacteria forming an apatite coating.

Andrei P. Sommer, Ph.D., University of Ulm, Central Institute of Biomedical Engineering, Ulm, Germany: Copublished with Kajander about nanobacteria and kidney stone formation and light-induced replication of nanobacteria. Expert in near-field optical analysis.

Eduardo Turcott, McGill University, Electron Microscopy Centre, Montreal, Canada: Coresearches nanobacteria in dental pulp.

Hojatollah Vali, Ph.D., Centre Director, McGill University Electron Microscopy Centre, Montreal, Canada: Researches nanobacteria and worked with David McKay and Neva Çiftçioğlu's team on investigating nanobes in a Martian meteorite. Copublished research on nanobacteria in dental pulp.

TESTING LABS

Many clinical labs are being used throughout the world to test for nanobacteria, but **Nanobac Oy,** based in Finland, is the pioneer. It was the first to develop tests for detecting nanobacteria. Its methods form the basis for methods that commercial labs use for detecting nanobacteria infections. It was started by Olavi Kajander and Neva Çiftçioğlu and is controlled by Nanobac Life Sciences, Tampa, Florida.

NANOBACTERIA CRITICS

Charles F. A. Bryce, Professor, Braids Education Consultants, Edinburgh, Scotland: Published a paper claiming that apatite crystals have been mistaken for nanobacteria.

John O. Cisar, Ph.D., National Institutes of Health, National Institute of Dental and Craniofacial Research, Oral Infection and Immunity Branch, Bethesda, Maryland, United States: Published research questioning the existence of nanobacteria as free living organisms.

Elmer M. Cranton, M.D., Family Practice Physician, Mount Rainier Clinic, Yelm, Washington, United States: IV chelation expert who challenges evidence that nanobacteria cause arteriosclerotic plaque.

Jouni Issakainen, Mycologist, Turku University Central Hospital, Turku, Finland: Sparked a public scientific fraud investigation against Olavi Kajander in Finland. Kajander was later unconditionally cleared when the investigating committee dismissed the claims as groundless.

Dennis J. Kopecko, Ph.D., Chief, Laboratory of Enteric and Sexually Transmitted Diseases, Food and Drug Administration, Rockville, Maryland, United States: Collaborated with Cisar on nanobacteria research. Says they found no credible molecular evidence to support the existence of nanobacteria.

Jack Maniloff, Professor of Microbiology and Immunology, University of Rochester, New York, United States: Researches evolution of microbial cells and viruses. Calls nanobacteria "the cold fusion of microbiology."

RELATED RESEARCH ON OTHER TYPES OF NANO-ORGANISMS SUCH AS NAN[N]OBACTERIA/ARCHAEAE/NANOBES

Robert L. Folk, Ph.D., Professor Emeritus, University of Texas, Department of Geological Sciences, Austin, Texas, United States: One of the first to describe nanoscale bacteria-like organisms in geological specimens. Years later he participated in a study by the Mayo Clinic and University of Texas in 2002 that confirmed the original discovery by Dr. László Puskás of nanobacteria in the arterial plaque that characterizes heart disease.

Brenda L. Kirkland, Ph.D., Mississippi State University, Strakville, Mississippi, United States: Geologist who works with and copublished with Robert Folk.

David McKay, Ph.D., NASA, Lyndon B. Johnson Space Center, Space and Life Science Directorate, Houston, Texas, United States: Director of a section of the Mars Program at NASA that focuses on potential life forms on Mars. Published a controversial paper showing evidence of life in a Martian meteorite. He brought the work of Neva Çiftçioğlu to the attention of NASA, after which she was invited by the agency to help it investigate nanobacteria.

Richard Y. Morita: First used the term "nannobacteria" with two *n*'s in a 1988 paper.[1] He has also written a book on nutrient-poor environments in which nano-bacteria may thrive.[2] This is a key to understanding how they survive.

Karl Stetter, Ph.D., Professor, University of Regensburg, Regensburg, Germany: Discovered *Nanoarchaeum equitans* in volcanic vents in Iceland that may be related to particles discovered years earlier by Robert Folk. Oversaw the ground-breaking sequencing of their DNA and identified the inability of standard tests to recognize some nucleic acids.

Philippa J. R. Uwins, Ph.D., Senior Research Fellow, University of Queensland, Centre for Microscopy and Microanalysis, St. Lucia, Australia: Along with col-leagues A. Taylor and R. Webb, published research on the discovery of "nanobes" and on the lower size limits of life. Uwins's team has resisted calling her discovery "nanobacteria." Instead they have given them the name "nanobes" until more is discovered and researched.

Milton Wainwright, Department of Molecular Biology and Biotechnology, University of Sheffield, Sheffield, United Kingdom: Wrote an article putting the discovery of nanobacteria in historical context, urging scientists to keep an open mind regarding the role of nanobacteria in human disease and cancer.

JOURNALISTS WHO HAVE COVERED NANOBACTERIA

Alison Abbott, Ph.D., Senior European Correspondent, *Nature* Magazine, Munich, Germany: Covers controversial stories in the field of genetics. Wrote stories in 1999 and 2000 about nanobacteria and the academic fraud accusation against Dr. Kajander.

Eric Berger, *Houston Chronicle*: Wrote a summary article on the nanobacteria discoveries and controversy with a focus on research being done at the Johnson Space Center in Houston.

Allan Hamilton, Ph.D., Professor, University of Aberdeen, Institute of Medical Sciences, Department of Molecular and Cell Biology, Aberdeen, United Kingdom: Produced a summary article on the debates exploring whether nanobacteria are alive or not.

Stephen Hart: Has written numerous informative articles on nanobacteria in *Astrobiology* magazine.

Jenny Hogan, *New Scientist*: Wrote one of the major summary articles on human nanobacteria discoveries and controversy in relation to heart disease.

Douglas Mulhall: Has written articles about human nanobacteria and was the first to discuss the nanobiotic treatment for nanobacteria in his book, *Our Molecular Future: How Nanotechnology, Robotics, Genetics, and Artificial Intelligence Will Transform Our World* (Amherst, NY: Prometheus Books, 2002).

Wayne P. Olson: Edited *Rapid Analytical Microbiology: The Chemistry and Physics of Microbial Identification (*Storrington West Sussex, UK: Sue Horwood Publishing, 2003), which includes a chapter about nanobacteria. Wrote a nanobacteria commentary in *PDA Journal of Pharmaceutical Sciences and Technology.*

Sonya Pemberton, Karena Slaninka, Filmmakers: Wrote, directed, and produced *Alien Underworld* (Tattooed Media, 2002), one of the first televised documentaries about nanobacteria. First broadcast in Australia.

Cynthia Smoot, FOX TV reporter in Tampa, Florida, United States: Produced a documentary on nanobiotics featuring Mezo, Kajander, and Maniscalco.

Michael Ray Taylor: Published what is arguably the first book about nanobacteria: *Dark Life: Martian Nanobacteria, Rock Eating Cave Bugs and Other Extreme Organisms of Inner Earth and Outer Space* (New York: Scribner, 1999).

INSURANCE

Alan Iezzi, M.D., F.A.A.F.P., Founder, Patient Directed Care, Tampa, Florida, United States: Medical director of a company with a program to let patients select their own treatments based on a discount system that removes insurers from making decisions for patients and doctors. Plans to include nanobiotics in the program.

SOME PRACTICING PHYSICIANS

Patrick Fratellone, M.D., F.A.C.C., Executive Medical Director of The Fratellone Group for Integrative Cardiology and Medicine, New York, New York, United States: Medical practice focuses on two epidemics: diabetes and obesity. Participated in the first NanobacTX-ACES Multicenter Study. Participated in a study of nanobiotic treatment in cardiac patients with diabetes.

Benedict S. Maniscalco, M.D., F.A.C.C., Tampa, Florida, United States: One of America's leading cardiologists who supervised the first formal clinical study of heart patients taking nanobiotics, the NanobacTX-ACES II.

James C. Roberts Jr., M.D., F.A.C.C., Comprehensive Heart Care—EECP Center of Northwest Ohio, Toledo, United States: An experienced practitioner of EECP therapy, which is described in this book. One of the first cardiologists to prescribe nanobiotics. His Web site (http://www.heartfixer.com) contains among the most comprehensive independent analyses available to the public. Participated in the NanobacTX-ACES Multicenter Study.

Daniel A. Shoskes, M.D., F.R.C.S., Director of Renal Transplant, Cleveland Clinic Florida, Department of Urology, Weston, Florida, United States: Has written leading papers on the role of biofilm and calcification in prostatitis. He is also investigating potential impacts of nanobiotics on disease in patients.

Stephen Sinatra, M.D., F.A.C.C., F.A.C.N., New England Heart and Longevity Center, Manchester, Connecticut, United States: One of the pioneering physicians who prescribed nanobiotics.

Daniel N. Tucker, M.D., Allergist and Immunologist, West Palm Beach, Florida, United States: Prescribing physician who is optimistic about the nanobiotic treatment but reserves judgment on what exactly nanobacteria may prove to be.

How Nanobacteria May Trigger the Atherosclerotic Process

T his "plain language" outline of the role of nanobacteria in atherosclerosis was written in consultation with Neva Çiftçioğlu, Olavi Kajander, Benedict Maniscalco, and Gary Mezo. It is a "work in progress" that may constitute the beginnings of a unifying theory of how coronary and other types of heart disease develop.

There are many possible pathways for nanobacteria to enter the human body. Here is a sequence where nanobacteria enter the body via contaminated vaccines, blood transfusions, contaminated water, or other possible sources. The process described below may take years or decades:

1. Nanobacteria enter the bloodstream directly or pass through the digestive system. They are carried throughout the capillaries, veins, and arteries. They replicate once every three to six days and grow by using calcium, phosphate, and lipids available in the blood.

2. At this stage the body can still get rid of many nanobacteria. They are excreted harmlessly into the urine. However, a few may get stuck in the kidney filtration system walls. Others are carried in the blood and get stuck in arteries and veins where flow is reduced at a splitting, bend, or narrowing in capillary beds of tissue or at a site of injury or tumor growth.

3. As they grow, nanobacteria form colonies and secrete biofilm. The slimy biofilm helps nanobacteria work together as a group and get food. It also helps the colonies to invade healthy cells. Later, it will help to build a hard protective shell. The multiple roles of this biofilm as a smokescreen, toxin, and defense are specific to nanobacteria.

4. Nanobacteria cause death to cells that internalize them. It is believed by the researchers that the human body has only a limited capacity to kill them. It tries to wall them off, but this only slows their growth when they are in calcified form and may also exacerbate the process of calcification. As the colony grows, signs of persistent infection arise and the body's defenses go into more aggressive action. White blood cells begin to attack the colony. They are triggered by the presence of toxins generated by nanobacteria and by inflammatory signals from cells. This is accelerated by premature death of cells from invasion of the nanobacteria. In response to the white blood cell attacks, nanobacteria shield themselves by secreting more slimy biofilm. Fatty streaks form on this battlefield as a by-product of the "inflammatory cascade" response. This is an extraordinarily complex process.

5. The body surrounds the area of nanobacterial infection much in the same way that it does with a cyst. The available nutrient supply for the nanobacteria begins to diminish. This is where a special property of nanobacteria comes into play. The colonies secrete calcium phosphate to build a sticky slime that hardens into an igloo-like shell that encases them. One shell can grow to be about two to three microns in diameter and may contain several specialized "mother" units. These may later spin off thousands of smaller nanobacteria known as "buds." Millions of shells aggregate to form calcified deposits that over time will be visible and quantifiable on a rapid CT scan.

6. The encased nanobacteria go into semihibernation but continue to grow their shells and also produce buds of tiny nanobacteria. Thus, the calcium deposit continues to grow upon itself "coral-like." This process occurs more slowly than replication of unencased nanobacteria, but it still continues relentlessly.

7. At this point, nanobacteria can be found in different stages throughout the body: growing, replicating, secreting biofilm, semihibernating in shells, and producing buds while being calcified and walled off within arteries and veins.

8. Meanwhile, the wall of the artery where the nanobacteria colony is located has been swelling in an inflammatory response to this infection. An inflammatory response occurs when tissues are injured by bacteria, toxins, or another cause. Damaged tissue releases chemicals that cause blood vessels to leak fluid and stimulate localized swelling. This helps to isolate the foreign substance from further contact with body tissues. The inflammatory response also attracts an invasion of "host cells" to the area. Together, these processes initiate the formation of a complex group of fatty, fibrous, and calcified deposits, otherwise referred to as

"plaque." The calcified deposits in atherosclerotic plaques form about 20 percent of this mass.

9. After many years, the growing plaque reduces the diameter of blood vessels. As our immune system continues to try to clean up the infection, the composition of the plaque changes. The relative amount of soft plaque decreases while "hard" plaque generated by nanobacterial calcification increases. At the same time, the body tries to bore new blood vessels into the plaque. Inadvertently, this feeds more nutrients to the semidormant nanobacteria, reviving them and causing their activity to accelerate, resulting in new inflammatory responses.

10. The process of nanobacteria replication repeats itself in many more locations. Deposits may form in the kidneys to trigger kidney stones or in the eyes to build cataracts. They may lodge in the muscles or joints to initiate arthritis-like or fibromyalgia-like symptoms.

11. This massive invasion triggers a chronic inflammatory response throughout the body, sending the immune system into a lifelong overdrive that ultimately will cause a crisis.

12. Eventually an artery clogs, or the artery wall ruptures as it becomes brittle, then stretches, causing a clot that leads to death or heart failure. Clotting is a problem because nanobacteria seem to bind together with prothrombin, the chemical that generates clots.

13. If a surgical procedure such as angioplasty is used on blood vessels, it releases billions of nanobacteria when their shelters are "smashed" and the nanobacteria are exposed to nutrient-rich blood again. This kickstarts their cycle, causing an acute "inflammatory cascade." They begin to replicate rapidly. The body's defenses cannot cope, and a crisis may occur.

Bibliography

For information on additional papers aside from those shown here, please refer to the Notes section, which, in some cases, includes Web sites where the papers can be located.

ACADEMIC RESEARCH PAPERS

Ackerman, K., I. Kuronen, and E. O. Kajander. "Scanning Electron Microscopy of Nanobacteria—Novel Biofilm Producing Organisms in Blood." *Scanning* 15, no. III (1993).

Breitschwerdt, E., S. Sontakke, A. Cannedy, S. Hancock, and J. Bradley. "Infection with *Bartonella weissii* and Detection of *Nanobacterium sanguineum* Antigens in a North Carolina Beef Herd." *Journal of Clinical Microbiology* 39, no. 3 (March 2001): 879–82.

Bryce, Charles F. A. "Alternative View on the Putative Organism, *Nanobacterium sanguineum*." Braids Education Consultants, Edinburgh EH106NZ, Scotland (undated), http://www.heartfixer.com/Nanobacterium-Report.htm (accessed January 23, 2003).

Carr, S., A. Farb, W. Pearce, et al. "Activated Inflammatory Cells Are Associated with Plaque Rupture in Carotid Artery Stenosis." *Surgery* 122 (1997): 757–63.

Çiftçioğlu, N., and E. O. Kajander. "Interaction of Nanobacteria with Cultured Mammalian Cells." *Pathophysiology* 4 (1998): 259–70.

Çiftçioğlu, N., M. A. Miller-Hjelle, J. T. Hjelle, and E. O. Kajander. "Inhibition of Nanobacteria by Antimicrobial Drugs As Measured by a Modified Microdilution Method." *Antimicrobial Agents and Chemotherapy* 46 (July 2002): 2077–86.

Çiftçioğlu, Neva, David S. McKay, and E. Olavi Kajander. "Association between Nanobacteria and Periodontal Disease." *Circulation* 108 (August 2003): 58–59.

Cisar, John O., De-Qi Xu, John Thompson, William Swaim, Lan Hu, and Dennis J. Kopecko. "An Alternative Interpretation of Nanobacteria-Induced Biomineralization." *Proceedings of the National Academy of Sciences* 97 (October 10, 2000): 11511–15.

Freimuth, V., H. Linnan, and P. Polyxeni. "Communicating the Threat of Emerging Infections to the Public." *CDC Emerging Infectious Diseases* 6, no. 4 (2000).

Garcia-Cuerpo, E., E. O. Kajander, N. Çiftçioğlu, F. Lovaco-Castellano, et al. "Nanobacteria: An Experimental Neo-lithogenesis Model." *Arch Esp Urol* 53, no. 4 (May 2000): 291–303.

Greenwald, R. "Treatment of Destructive Arthritic Disorders with MMP Inhibitors." *Ann NY Acad Sci* 732 (1994): 199–205.

Hjelle, T., M. Miller-Hjelle, I. Poxton, E. O. Kajander, N. Çiftçioğlu, et al. "Endotoxin and Nanobacteria in Polycystic Kidney Disease." *International Society of Nephrology; Kidney International* 57 (2000): 2360–74.

Holvoet, P., et al. "Circulating Oxidized LDL a Sensitive Marker of CAD." *Arterioscler Thromb Vasc Biol* 21 (2001): 844–48.

Houpikian, Pierre, and Didier Raoult. "Traditional and Molecular Techniques for the Study of Emerging Bacterial Diseases: One Laboratory's Perspective." *Emerging Infectious Diseases* 8, no. 2 (February 2002).

Jantos, C., A. Nesseler, W. Waas, et al. "Low Prevalence of *Chlamydia pneumoniae* in Atherectomy Specimens from Patients with Coronary Heart Disease." *Clin Infect Dis* 28, no. 5 (1999): 988–92.

Jelic, T. M., A. M. Malas, S. S. Groves, B. Jin, P. F. Mellen, G. Osborne, R. Roque, J. G. Rosencrance, and H. H. Chang. "Nanobacteria-Caused Mitral Valve Calciphylaxis in a Man with Diabetic Renal Failure." *South Med J* 97, no. 2 (February 2004): 194–98.

Joseph, A., D. Ackerman, J. Talley, et al. "Manifestations of Coronary Atherosclerosis in Young Trauma Victims: An Autopsy Study." *J Am Coll Cardiol* 22 (1993): 459–67.

Kajander, E. O., K. Aho, and V. Segal. "Apatite Biofilm Forming Agent: Nanobacteria as a Model System for Biomineralization and Biological Standard for NOA: A Preliminary Study." *Proceedings of the 2nd International Conference on Near-Field Optical Analysis: Photodynamic Therapy and Photobiology Effects*, Houston, TX (30.05.–01.06.01). NASA/CP 210786 (October 2002): 51–57.

Kajander, E. O., N. Çiftçioğlu, K. Aho, and E. Garcia-Cuerpo. "Characteristics of Nanobacteria and Their Possible Role in Stone Formation." Invited Editorial. *Urol Res* 31, no. 2 (June 2003): 47–54.

Kajander, E. O., N. Çiftçioğlu, M. Miller-Hjelle, and T. Hjelle. "Nanobacteria: Controversial Pathogens in Nephrolithiasis and Polycystic Kidney Disease." *Current Opinion Nephrology and Hypertension* 10 (May 2001): 445–52.

Khullar, M., S. K. Sharma, S. K. Singh, P. Bajwa, F. A. Sheikh, V. Relan, and M. Sharma. "Morphological and Immunological Characteristics of Nanobacteria from Human Renal Stones of a North Indian Population." *Urol Res* 32, no. 3 (June 2004): 190–95.

Kweider, M., G. Lowe, G. Murray, D. Kinane, and D. McGowan. "Dental Disease, Fibrinogen and White Cell Count: Links with Myocardial Infarction." *Scottish Med J* 38, no. 3 (June 1993): 73–74.

Li, Y., Y. Wen, Z. Yang, H. Wei, W. Liu, A. Tan, X. Wu, Q. Wang, S. Huang, E. O. Kajander, and N. Çiftçioğlu. "Culture and Identification of Nanobacteria in Bile." [In Chinese.] *Zhonghua Yi Xue Za Zhi* 25 (2002): 1557–60. In this work, 61 percent of seventy-five patient bile samples removed during cholecystectomy were positive for nanobacteria with culture and TEM and with a novel calcification assay.

Libby, P., D. Egan, and S. Skarlatos. "Roles of Infectious Agents in Atherosclerosis and Restenosis." *Circulation* 96 (1997): 4095–103.

Lieske, John C., Vivek Kumar, Gerard Farell-Baril, Shihui Yu, Jon E. Charlesworth, Ewa Rzewuska-Lech, Peter LaBreche, Sandra R. Severson, and Virginia M. Miller. "Detection and Propagation of Calcified Nanostructures from Human Aneurysms," *JACC Abstract Book* 43, no. 5 (March 2004) 1059–13: p. 13A.

Lopez-Brea, M., and R. Selgas. "Nanobacteria as a Cause of Renal Diseases and Vascular Calcifying Pathology in Renal Patients ('Endovascular Lithiasis')." *Enferm Infec Microbiol Clin* 18, no. 10 (December 2000): 491–92.

Maniscalco, B. S., and K. A. Taylor. "Calcification in Coronary Artery Disease Can Be Reversed by EDTA–Tetracycline Long-Term Chemotherapy." *Pathophysiology* DOI:10.1016/j.pathophys.2004.06.001 (accepted June 3, 2004).

Miller, V. M., G. Rodgers, J. A. Charlesworth, B. Kirkland, S. R. Severson, T. E. Rasmussen, M. Yagubyan, J. C. Rodgers, F. R. Cockerill, R. L. Folk, V. Kumar, G. Farell-Baril, and J. C. Lieske. "Evidence of Nanobacterial-like Structures in Human Calcified Arteries and Cardiac Valves." *Am J Physiol Heart Circ Physiol* 287, no. 3 (September 2004): H1115–24.

Miller-Hjelle, M. A., J. T. Hjelle, N. Çiftçioğlu, and E. O. Kajander. "Nanobacteria: Methods for Growth and Identification of This Recently Discovered Calciferous Agent. In *Rapid Analytical Microbiology: The Chemistry and Physics of Microbial Identification*. Ed. W. Olson. Storrington West Sussex, UK: Sue Horwood Publishing, 2003.

Nazir, R., and S. Gupta. "Clinical Significance of Coronary Calcification." *Emer Med* (February 2001): 107–10.

O'Rourke, R. A., et al. "American College of Cardiology/American Heart Association Expert Consensus Document on Electronbeam Computed Tomography for Diagnosis and Prognosis of Coronary Artery Disease." *J Am Coll Cardiol* 36 (2000): 326.

Pasterkamp, G., A. Schoneveld, A. C. van del Wal, et al. "Inflammation of the Atherosclerotic Cap and Shoulder of the Plaque Is a Common and Locally

Observed Feature in Unruptured Plaques of Femoral and Coronary Arteries." *Arterioscler Thromb Vasc Biol* 19 (1999): 54–58.

Ray, J., and W. Stetler-Stevenson. "The Role of Matrix Metalloproteinases and Their Inhibitors in Tumor Invasion, Metastasis and Angiogenesis." *Eur Res J* 7 (1994): 2062–72.

Rifai, N., R. Joubran, H. Yu, et al. "Inflammatory Markers in Men with Angiographically Documented Coronary Heart Disease." *Clin Chem* 45 (1999): 1967–73.

Rumberger, J., D. Simons, L. Fitzpatrick, et al. "Coronary Artery Calcium Area by Electron Beam Computed Tomography and Coronary Atherosclerotic Plaque Area: A Histopathologic Correlative Study." *Circulation* 92 (1995): 2157–62.

Sangiorgi, G., J. Rumberger, A. Severson, et al. "Arterial Calcification and NOT Lumen Stenosis Is Highly Correlated with Atherosclerotic Plaque Burdens in Humans: A Histologic Study of 723 Coronary Artery Segments Using Nondecalcifying Methodology." *J Am Coll Cardiol* 31 (1998): 126–33.

Sedivy, R., and W.B. Battistutti. "Nanobacteria Promote Crystallization of Psammoma Bodies in Ovarian Cancer." *APMIS* 111, no. 10 (October 2003): 951–54.

Sommer, A. P., H. Hassinen, and E. O. Kajander. "Light Induced Replication of Nanobacteria—A Preliminary Report." *J Clin Laser Med Surg* 20 (2002): 241–44.

Sommer, A. P., and E. O. Kajander. "Nanobacteria-Induced Kidney Stone Formation: Novel Paradigm Based on the FERMIC Model." *Crystal Growth and Design* 2 (2002): 563–65.

Sommer, A. P., David S. McKay, Neva Çiftçioğlu, Uri Oron, Adam R. Mester, and E. Olavi Kajander. "Living Nanovesicles: Chemical and Physical Survival Strategies of Primordial Biosystems; Living Nanovesicles Perspectives." *Journal of Proteome Research* 2, no. 4 (July/August 2003): 441–43.

Sommer, A. P., U. Oron, E. O. Kajander, and A. R. Mester. "Stressed Cells Survive Better with Light." *Journal of Proteome Research* 1 (2002): 475.

Vainshtein, M., and E. Kudriashova. "Nanobacteria." *Mikrobiologiia* 69, no. 2 (2000): 163–74.

van der Wal, A. C., A. Becker, C. M. van der Loos, et al. "Site of Intimal Rupture or Erosion of Thrombosed Coronary Atherosclerotic Plaques Is Characterized by an Inflammatory Process Irrespective of the Dominant Plaque Morphology." *Circulation* 89 (1994): 36–44.

Wen, Y., Y. G. Li, Z. L. Yang, X. J. Wang, H. Wei, W. Liu, A. L. Tan, X. Y. Miao, Q. W. Wang, S. F. Huang, E. O. Kajander, and N. Çiftçioğlu. "Nanobacteria in Serum, Bile and Gallbladder Mucosa of Cholecystolithiasis Patients." [In Chinese.] *Zhonghua Wai Ke Za Zhi* 41, no. 4 (April 2003): 267–70.

BOOKS

Most of the information for this book was gleaned from scientific publications, subject interviews, and correspondence rather than books because while thousands of books deal with heart disease and cancer or diets to prevent them, relatively few deal with pathological calcification. Many books that deal with such calcification are out of date, out of print, or inaccessible to lay readers. The authors also scanned dozens of diet books for mentions of "calcification," but we do not list most of them here since they do not contain relevant information about pathological calcification, its cause, or a possible remedy. Therefore, the list in this section is short.

Agatston, Arthur. *The South Beach Diet: The Delicious, Doctor-Designed, Foolproof Plan for Fast and Healthy Weight Loss.* New York: Rodale Press, 2003.

Atkins, Robert C. *Dr. Atkins' New Diet Revolution.* New York: Avon Books, 1999 (revised 2003).

Beers, Mark H., and Robert Berkow, eds. *The Merck Manual of Diagnosis and Therapy*, 17th ed., Centennial Ed., Whitehouse Stn., NJ: Merck Research Laboratories, 1999. [This manual has been updated online in 2004.]

Dvonch, Louis A., and Russell Dvonch. *The Heart Attack Germ.* New York: Writer's Showcase, 2003.

Garcia-Cuerpo, E. *Litogenesis: Estado de la Investigacion.* Barcelona: Publicaciones Permanyer, 2003.

Ewald, Paul W. *Evolution of Infectious Diseases.* New York: Oxford University Press, 1994.

Ewald, Paul W. *Plague Time: How Stealth Infections Cause Cancer, Heart Disease and Other Deadly Ailments.* New York: Anchor Books, 2002.

Garrett, Laurie. *Betrayal of Trust: The Collapse of Global Public Health.* New York: Hyperion, 2001.

Mulhall, Douglas. *Our Molecular Future: How Nanotechnology, Robotics, Genetics, and Artificial Intelligence Will Transform Our World.* Amherst, NY: Prometheus, 2002.

Null, Gary. *Seven Steps to Perfect Health.* Austin, TX: I Books, 2001.

Ornish, Dean. *Dr. Dean Ornish's Program for Reversing Heart Disease.* New York: Ballantine, 1992 (revised 2003).

Rath, Matthias. *Why Animals Don't Get Heart Attacks . . . But Humans Do!* Fremont, CA: MR Publishing Inc, 2003.

Taylor, Michael Ray. *Dark Life: Martian Nanobacteria, Rock-Eating Cave Bugs, and Other Extreme Organisms of Inner Earth and Outer Space.* New York: Scribner, 1999.

HELPFUL WEB SITES

There are dozens of Web sites about calcification, nanobacteria, nanobes, and "nannobacteria" and thousands of Web sites on diseases related to them. Here are a few directory Web sites that lead to them. Please refer to Web sites shown in the Notes section for more information about specific calcification-related illnesses.

http://www.astrobio.net—Home page of *Astrobiology* magazine, which has occasional articles on nanobacteria.

http://www.calcify.com—Home page for this book. Provides updates to information from the book, supplementary data, links to other Web sites, and reviews of the book. The site changes often as information becomes available.

http://en.wikipedia.org/wiki/Nanobacteria—Web encyclopedia entry for nanobacteria with links to articles.

http://www.heartfixer.com/indexNB.htm—Nanobacteria section of the Web site of Ohio-based Dr. James C. Roberts, one of the first cardiologists to prescribe nanobiotics. Valuable case studies. To find this site if the address changes, do a Web search for his name.

http://www.lifescore.com/nanoscore.htm—Home page of a San Diego–based clinic offering treatment for nanobacteria infections.

http://www.microscopy-uk.org.uk/nanobes/nanoimages.html—Images and links of nanobes listed on the Microscopy UK portal.

http://www.noaw.com/Nanobacteria/nanobacteria.htm—Nanobacteria section of Network for Effective Women's Services (NEWS) based in Watkinsville, Georgia. Has a good summary of links to nanobacteria Web sites.

http://www.nanobac.com—Home page of Nanobac Oy, a European subsidiary of Nanobac Life Sciences. Based in Kuopio, Finland. Developed the diagnostics for nanobacteria.

http://www.nanobaclifesciences.com—Home page of Nanobac Life Sciences in Tampa, Florida, the company that researches nanobiotics and test supplies for detecting nanobacteria.

http://www.nanobacsciences.com—Home page of Nanobac Sciences, which distributes a nanobiotic nutraceutical.

http://www.thenanotechnologygroup.org/id71.htm—Web page with a case history as told by a cataract patient.

http://www.uq.edu.au/nanoworld/uwins.html—Web page of Dr. Philippa Uwins at the University of Queensland in Australia that describes the geological forms that she has named "nanobes." Has good links to other stories.

Notes

CHAPTER I: YOU'RE ON THE CALCIFICATION LIST

1. "Calcification–the process by which organic tissue becomes hardened by a deposit of calcium salts within its substance." MerckSource Dorland's Illustrated Medical Dictionary, http://www.mercksourcompp/ucns/ns_hl_dorlands .jspzQzpgzEzzSzppdocszSzuszSzcomm | onzSzdorlandszSzdorlandzSzdmd_c _02zPz.htm (accessed April 25, 2004).

2. "Breast Implant Risks," FDA, Center for Devices and Radiological Health, November 2000, http://www.fda.gov/cdrh/breastimplants/breast_implant _risks_brochure.html (accessed March 25, 2004).

3. Daniel H. Solomon, Elizabeth W. Karlson, Eric B. Rimm, Carolyn C. Cannuscio, Lisa A. Mandl, JoAnn E. Manson, Meir J. Stampfer, and Gary C. Curhan, "Cardiovascular Morbidity and Mortality in Women Diagnosed with Rheumatoid Arthritis," *Circulation* 107 (March 11, 2003): 1303–7.

4. "Astronauts Risk Kidney Stones," BBC, November 8, 2001, http://news.bbc .co.uk/1/hi/health/1643632.stm (accessed February 15, 2003). Also, "Renal Stone Risk during Space Flight: Assessment and Countermeasure Validation," *NASA Fact Sheet*, July 2001, http://www1.msfc.nasa.gov/NEWSROOM/ background/facts/renal.html (accessed February 15, 2003).

5. E. M. Reiman, K. Chen, G. E. Alexander, R. J. Caselli, D. Bandy, A. Prouty, and C. Burns, "Abnormalities in Regional Brain Activity in Young Adults at Genetic Risk for Late-Onset Alzheimer's Disease," Abstract presentation at the 8th International Conference on Alzheimer's Disease and Related Disorders, Stockholm, 2002, http://www.alz.washington.edu/NONMEMBER/ PDF/azadc2.pdf (accessed April 17, 2004).

6. "Alzheimer's Disease," Duke University Medical Center, Psychiatry and Behavioral Sciences, http://psychiatry.mc.duke.edu/CMRIS/ED/Alzheimers.htm (accessed January 23, 2004).

7. "It can also show calcium deposits, which are present in some types of brain tumors." "Brain Tumor," MedicineNet Diseases and Conditions, http://www .medicinenet.com/Brain_Tumor/page3.htm (accessed April 25, 2004).

8. "Cranial Calcification," Medline Plus Encyclopedia, National Institutes of Health, January 10, 2003, http://www.nlm.nih.gov/medlineplus/ency/ imagepages/9228.htm (accessed March 30, 2004).

9. Some studies show a link between the pineal gland and MS. "PC [pineal calcification] was seen in 100% of MS patients . . . In the control sample, PC was found in 42.8% . . . Thus, the strikingly high prevalence of PC in MS provides indirect support for an association between MS and ab- normalities of the pineal gland." R. Sandyk and G. I. Awerbuch, "The Pineal Gland in Multiple Sclerosis," *Int J Neurosci* 61, no. 1–2 (Novem- ber 1991): 61–67 abstract, http://www.ncbi.nlm.nih.gov/entrez/query.fcgi ?cmd=Retrieve&db=pubmed&dopt=Abstract&list_uids=1809735 (ac- cessed April 25, 2004).

10. "Clinical Guidelines for the Care of Patients with Tuberous Sclerosis Complex," Tuberous Sclerosis Association, http://www.tuberous-sclerosis .org/professionals/guidelines.shtml (accessed January 23, 2004).

11. "Cancer Facts," National Institutes of Health, http://cis.nci.nih.gov/fact/5 _6.htm (accessed February 10, 2004).

12. "Mammogram Calcifications," Medline Plus, National Institutes of Health, http://www.nlm.nih.gov/medlineplus/ency/article/002113.htm (accessed Janu- ary 23, 2004).

13. "Breast Implant Risks," FDA, Center for Devices and Radiological Health, November 2000, http://www.fda.gov/cdrh/breastimplants/breast_implant _risks_brochure.html (accessed April 25, 2004).

14. James H. Bedino, "*Mycobacterium tuberculosis*: An In-Depth Discussion for Embalmers Part 2," *Expanding Encyclopedia of Mortuary Practices* 637 (1999), http://www.champion-newera.com/CHAMP.PDFS/encyclo637.pdf (accessed April 26, 2004).

15. "Arthritis," National Center for Chronic Disease Prevention, http://www.cdc .gov/nccdphp/arthritis/index.htm (accessed January 13, 2004).

16. "Ankylosing Spondylitis: Exams and Tests," WebMD, http://my.webmd.com/ hw/arthritis/tr4515.asp?lastselectedguid={5FE84E90-BC77-4056-A91C- 9531713CA348} (accessed March 15, 2004).

17. "Bone Spurs," Spine-health.com, http://www.spine-health.com/topics/cd/ spurs/spurs01.html (accessed February 10, 2004).

18. "What Does Bone Cancer Look Like on an X-ray?" Cancer Research UK, http://www.cancerhelp.org.uk/help/default.asp?page=386 (accessed April 25, 2004).

19. "Bursitis and Tendon Injury: Exams and Tests," WebMD, http://my.webmd .com/hw/health_guide_atoz/n3752.asp?lastselectedguid={5FE84E90-BC77- 4056-A91C-9531713CA348} (accessed April 5, 2004).

20. "Bone Formation and Calcification in Cardiovascular Disease," National Institutes of Health, January 2, 2001, http://grants2.nih.gov/grants/guide/rfa- files/RFA-HL-01-014.html (accessed March 29, 2004). Also, "New Evidence

Connecting Cardiovascular Disease and Osteoporosis," National Institute of Arthritis and Musculoskeletal and Skin Diseases, NIAMS-NHLBI Working Group September 14–15, 1999, Bethesda, Maryland, http://www.niams.nih .gov/ne/reports/sci_wrk/1999/bnhrtsm.htm (accessed April 3, 2004).

21. "Treatment for Vertigo May Provide Effective, Nonsurgical Relief for Ménière's Disease," News Release, American Academy of Otolaryngology Head and Neck Surgery, September 21, 2002, http://www.newswise.com/ articles/2002/9/MENIERES.AAO.html (accessed April 26, 2004). Also, Ivy M. Alexander, "The Spin on Dizziness," *Yale Healthcare Newsletter* II, no 6. (1999), http://www.yale.edu/yuhs/highlights/yhc/nov_dec99.pdf (accessed April 10, 2004). Also, information on calcification of inner ear stones provided in interview by the authors with E. Olavi Kajander, April 25, 2003.

22. "Calcification of lens" is a classification in "Ophthalmological Coding Manual," Intranet version, November 2001, http://www.vumc.nl/oogheelkunde/ Ophthalmological%20Coding%20Manual.pdf (accessed March 29, 2003).

23. "What Is Glaucoma?" Glaucoma Research Foundation, http://www.glaucoma .org/learn/ (accessed January 15, 2004).

24. "Macular Degeneration," Medline Plus Encyclopedia, National Institutes of Health, http://www.nlm.nih.gov/medlineplus/ency/article/001000 .htm#contentDescription (accessed January 15, 2004).

25. Calcification is found in Drusen deposits of macular degeneration. "Drusen deposits vary in size and may exist in a variety of forms from soft to calcified." Quote from "Age Related Macular Degeneration: ARMD: The Disease," Indiana University School of Optometry, http://www.opt.indiana.edu/clinics/ pt_educ/armd/disease.htm (accessed April 17, 2004).

26. Peter C. Buetow, James L. Buck, Norman J. Carr, and Linda Pantongrag-Brown, "Colorectal Adenocarcinoma: Radiologic-Pathologic Correlation," *RadioGraphics* 15, no. 1 (January 1, 1995), http://www.rsna.org/REG/publications/rg/afip/ privateM/1995/0015/0001/0127/1.htm (accessed April 25, 2004).

27. "Extraintestinal Complications of IBD," Crohn's and Colitis Foundation of America, http://www.ccfa.org/research/info/complications (accessed March 29, 2004).

28. "Kidney Stones," National Kidney and Urologic Diseases Information Clearinghouse, http://www.niddk.nih.gov/health/kidney/pubs/stonadul/stonadul .htm#what. Also, "Nephrolithiasis," Medline Plus Encyclopedia, National Institutes of Health, http://www.nlm.nih.gov/medlineplus/ency/article/000458 .htm (accessed January 13, 2004).

29. Aijaz Ahmed and Emmet B. Keeffe, "Gallstones and Biliary Tract Disease," in D. C. Dale and D. D. Federman, eds., *Scientific American Medicine* vol. 1, pt. 4, chap. 6 (New York: Scientific American): 1–11.

30. "What Are the Risk Factors for Gallbladder Cancer?" *American Cancer Society*, http://www.cancer.org/docroot/CRI/content/CRI_2_4_2X_What _are_the_risk_factors_for_gall_bladder_cancer_68.asp (accessed April 25, 2004).

31. "Addison's Disease," Medline Plus, National Institutes of Health, http://www .nlm.nih.gov/medlineplus/ency/article/000378.htm (accessed January 15, 2004). Also, telephone interview by the authors with E. Olavi Kajander, May 7, 2003, regarding kidney stones being a characteristic of Addison's disease.

32. "Hypoparathyroidism," Medline Plus Medical Encyclopedia, National Institutes of Health, http://www.nlm.nih.gov/medlineplus/ency/article/000385.htm (accessed January 13, 2004).

33. Laura Mauri, Mark Reisman, Maurice Buchbinder, Jeffrey J. Popma, Samin K. Sharma, Donald E. Cutlip, Kalon K.L. Ho, Ross Prpic, Peter J. Zimetbaum, and Richard E. Kuntz, "Comparison of Rotational Atherectomy with Conventional Balloon Angioplasty in the Prevention of Restenosis of Small Coronary Arteries: Results of the Dilatation vs Ablation Revascularization Trial Targeting Restenosis (DART)," *Am Heart J* 145, no. 5 (2003): 847–54, http://www.medscape.com/viewarticle/456231_print (accessed May 10, 2004). For insight into the cost implications of getting rid of restenosis in stents, see Ron Winslow, "New Stents a Boon for Patients May Affect Rising Health Costs," *Wall Street Journal,* December 24, 2002, p. 1.

34. Daniel Q. Haney, "More Children Getting Adult Diabetes," *Associated Press,* April 13, 2003, http://www.rednova.com/news/stories/2/2003/04/13/story002.html (accessed April 10, 2004).

35. Neal X. Chen and Sharon M. Moe, "Arterial Calcification in Diabetes," *Current Diabetes Reports* 3 (2003): 28–32 (February 1, 2003) abstract, http://www.biomedcentral.com/1534-4827/3/28/abstract (accessed April 10, 2004).

36. Peggy Lin, Lynne Goldberg, and Tania Phillips, "Calciphylaxis," *Wounds* 14, no. 5 (2002): 205–10, Medscape, http://www.medscape.com/viewarticle/438054 (accessed April 10, 2004).

37. G. C. Willis, "An Experimental Study of the Intimal Ground Substance in Atherosclerosis," *Canadian Medical Association Journal* (CMAJ) 69 (July 1953), http://www.internetwks.com/pauling/study.html (accessed April 3, 2004).

38. Federico Guercini, "Prostatitis 2000 Symptoms," http://www.prostatitis2000.org/eng/sintomatologia.htm (accessed April 28, 2004).

39. "Kidney Stones," National Kidney and Urologic Diseases Information Clearinghouse, http://www.niddk.nih.gov/health/kidney/pubs/stonadul/stonadul.htm#what. Also, "Nephrolithiasis," Medline Plus Encyclopedia, National Institutes of Health, http://www.nlm.nih.gov/medlineplus/ency/article/000458.htm (accessed January 13, 2004).

40. "Calcification is often found in uterine fibroids. Calcification is frequently present in benign and malignant ovarian tumors." Deborah Pate, "Common Intrapelvic Soft Tissue Calcification," *Roentgen Report*, http://www.chiroweb.com/archives/12/21/10.html (accessed April 25, 2004). Also, "Ovarian Fibroma," Medcyclopaedia Amersham Health, http://www.amershamhealth.com/medcyclopaedia/medical/Volume%20IV%202/OVARIAN%20FIBROMA.ASP (accessed April 25, 2004).

41. Philip Thomason, "Leiomyoma, Uterus (Fibroid)," eMedicine, January 11, 2002, http://www.emedicine.com/radio/topic777.htm (accessed April 25, 2004).

42. "Peyronie's Disease," National Kidney and Urologic Diseases Information Clearinghouse, *NIH Publication* No. 01-3902 (May 1995, updated September 2001), http://www.niddk.nih.gov/health/urolog/pubs/peyronie/peyronie.htm (accessed March 29, 2004).

43. Lisbeth Schjerling, Ebbe Kvist, Sven Grønvall Rasmussen and Anne Birthe Wåhlin, "Testicular Microlithiasis: The Necessity of Biopsy and Follow Up," *Ugeskr Læger* 164 (2002): 2041–45.

44. "Aging and the Skin: Normal Changes of Aging," *The Merck Manual of Geriatrics*, sec. 15, chap. 122, http://www.merck.com/mrkshared/mm _geriatrics/sec15/ch122.jsp (accessed April 25, 2004).

45. The protein is collagen. See "Scleroderma," Arthritis Foundation, http://www .arthritis.org/conditions/DiseaseCenter/scleroderma.asp (accessed January 17, 2004). Also, "Scleroderma," Amersham Health Encyclopedia, http://www .amershamhealth.com/medcyclopaedia/Volume%20III%201/scleroderma .asp (accessed January 17, 2004).

46. Susan Kinder Haake, "Microbiology of Dental Plaque," Periodontics Information Center, University of California, Los Angeles School of Dentistry, http://www.dent.ucla.edu/pic/members/microbio/mdphome.html (accessed March 29, 2004).

47. N. Çiftçioğlu, D. S. McKay, and E. O. Kajander, "Association between Nanobacteria and Periodontal Disease," *Circulation* 108 (August 2003): 58–59.

48. "Salivary Stones," MayoClinic.com, February 26, 2004, http://www.mayoclinic .com/invoke.cfm?id=HQ01323 (accessed April 23, 2004).

CHAPTER 2: WHEN THE TIMER STARTS TICKING

1. Malcolm East, "Life, Death and Calcium," University of Southampton, March 2002, chembytes e-zine, The Royal Society of Chemistry, http://www.chemsoc .org/chembytes/ezine/2002/east_mar02.htm (accessed March 29, 2004). Also, "Imbalances of calcium can lead to many health problems and excess calcium in nerve cells can cause their death." Quote from "Calcium," Cancerweb Dictionary, May 22, 1997, http://cancerweb.ncl.ac.uk/cgi-bin/omd?calcium (accessed January 15, 2004).

2. "Endocrine Control of Calcium and Phosphate Homeostasis," Hypertexts for Biomedical Sciences, Pathophysiology, Endocrine System, Colorado State University, http://arbl.cvmbs.colostate.edu/hbooks/pathphys/endocrine/ thyroid/calcium.html (accessed August 20, 2004).

3. "Dystrophic calcification: the deposition of calcium in abnormal tissue, such as scar tissue or atherosclerotic plaques, but without abnormalities of blood calcium." MerckSource Dorland's Illustrated Medical Dictionary, http://www .mercksource.com/pp/us/cns/cns_hl_dorlands.jspzQzpgzEzzSzppdocszSzu szSzcommonzSzdorlandszSzdorlandzSzdmd_c_02zPzhtm (accessed April 25, 2004).

4. "[W]e aren't sure what the healthiest or safest amount of dietary calcium is . . . In particular, these studies have reported that calcium doesn't actually appear to lower a person's risk for osteoporosis . . ." "Calcium and Milk," Harvard School of Public Health, http://www.hsph.harvard.edu/nutritionsource/ calcium.html (accessed April 25, 2004).

5. One drug company Web site says, "It's very difficult to get too much calcium. Any excess which the body cannot use is excreted from the body in the urine and stool. Daily consumption up to 2,500 mg has been shown to be safe." Calcium 101 GlaxoSmithKline, http://www.calciuminfo.com/pages/1_5faq .htm (accessed April 25, 2004).

6. "Drug-free Way to Drop High Blood Pressure: Cut Calories, Add Exercise," Press Release, Report to the Annual Meeting of the American Heart Association, Chicago, September 24, 2001, http://www.americanheart.org/presenter .jhtml?identifier=10993 (accessed January 20, 2004).

7. "Calcium Scan Predicts Heart Attack Risk in Physically Fit People," *American Heart Association Journal Report*, January 3, 2001, http://www.americanheart .org/presenter.jhtml?identifier=3292 (accessed April 3, 2004). The study authors, Irwin M. Feuerstein, M.D., Michael P. Brazaitis, M.D., Mark A. Vaitkus, Ph.D., and William F. Barko, M.D., found that there is no apparent link between calcification and fitness level. "We were surprised by the high (calcium) scores in a group that was very physically fit and had undergone routine physical examinations," said Jerel M. Zoltick, M.D., a U.S. Army cardiologist and consultant with the Office of the Surgeon General.

8. "Calcium," Chemical Elements.com, http://www.chemicalelements.com/ elements/ca.html (accessed January 1, 2004).

9. "Apatite," Moh's Hardness Scale, Simon Fraser University Department of Archaeology, http://www.sfu.ca/archaeology/museum/rock_id/mohs%20scale .html (accessed March 29, 2004).

10. "Basic Calcium Phosphate and Other Crystal Disorders," *The Merck Manual of Diagnosis and Therapy*, sec. 5, Musculoskeletal and Connective Tissue Disorders, chap. 55, Crystal-Induced Conditions, http://www.merck.com/ mrkshared/mmanual/section5/chapter55/55d.jsp (accessed March 1, 2004).

11. Y. Sun, X. R. Zeng, L. Wenger, and H. S. Cheung, "Basic Calcium Phosphate Crystals Stimulate the Endocytotic Activity of Cells: Inhibition by Anti-calcification Agents," *Biochem Biophys Res Commun* 312, no. 4 (December 2003): 1053–59. Also, G. M. McCarthy, J. A. Augustine, A. S. Baldwin, P. A. Christopherson, H. S. Cheung, P. R. Westfall, and R. I. Scheinman, "Molecular Mechanism of Basic Calcium Phosphate Crystal-Induced Activation of Human Fibroblasts," *J Biol Chem* 273, no. 52 (December 25, 1998): 35161–69.

12. Dennis Carson, "An Infectious Origin of Extraskeletal Calcification," *Proceedings of the National Academy of Sciences (PNAS)* 95, no. 14 (July 7, 1998): 7846–47.

13. We attribute this term to E. Olavi Kajander, who has used it in interviews with the authors.

14. "Small Blood Vessels Big Role Found," BBC, December 30, 2002, http://news .bbc.co.uk/2/hi/health/2609469.stm (accessed January 15, 2004). Also, Matthew C. P. Glyn, John G. Lawrenson, and Barbara J. Ward, "A Rho-Associated Kinase Mitigates Reperfusion-Induced Change in the Shape of Cardiac Capillary Endothelial Cells in Situ," *Journal of Cardiovascular Research* 57, no. 1 (2003): 195–206, http://www.escardiocontent.org/periodicals/ carres/article/PIIS0008636302006168/fulltext (accessed March 15, 2004).

15. Search results for the term "calcification," http://www.intelihealth.com (accessed May 9, 2004).

16. For example, when a patient asked about calcification of the optic nerve, known as "Drusen," the advising physician noted, "Unfortunately, I know of no treatment for this when it happens." Don Carl Bienfang, "Ask the Expert," Intellihealth, October 22, 2002, http://www.intelihealth.com/

IH/ihtIH?d=dmtATD&c=356533&p=~br,IHW|~st,24479|~r,WSIH
W000|~b,*| (accessed April 17, 2004). Responses by experts regarding
spinal stenosis also had no suggestions other than surgery for removing
calcium deposits. See http://www.intelihealth.com/IH/ihtIH?d=dmtATD
&c=353582&p=~br,IHW|~st,24479|~r,WSIHW000|~b,*| (accessed
April 17, 2004).

17. Johns Hopkins Arthritis Radiology Rounds states that "the cause of calcinosis
cutis is unknown." *Radiology Rounds*, round 7, http://www.hopkins-arthritis
.som.jhmi.edu/radrds/radiology_7/7_radrds_diagnosis.html (accessed April
17, 2004).

18. A good summary of contemporary thinking on this is Paul W. Ewald, *Plague
Time: How Stealth Infections Cause Cancers, Heart Disease and Other Deadly
Ailments* (New York: Anchor Books, 2002).

19. "CT Artery Scan at Rhode Island Hospital," http://www.lifespan.org/SvcLines/
CardiacSvcs/Diagnosis/CTartery.htm (accessed May 10, 2004).

20. Web site of the American Heart Association, http://www.heartcenteronline
.com/myheartdr/common/artprn_rev.cfm?filename=&ARTID=191
(accessed April 18, 2004).

21. Word search for "calcification" using http://www.google.com (accessed August
15, 2004).

22. Ibid. Word search using "cause of calcification."

23. Martin Bendszus, "Brain Damage after Surgical and Angio-graphic Heart
Procedures," *Geriatric Times* IV, no. 1 (January/February 2003), http://www
.geriatrictimes.com/g030231.html (accessed March 29, 2004).

24. Winslow, "New Stents a Boon for Patients May Affect Rising Health Costs,"
Wall Street Journal, December 24, 2002, p. 1.

25. Ibid.

26. "Extracorporeal Shock Wave Lithotripsy for the Treatment of Gallstones,
Pancreatic Stones and Bile Duct Stones," *The Regence Group Medical Policy
Manual*, approved date May 7, 2002, http://www.regence.com/trgmedpol/
surgery/sur81.html (accessed January 27, 2004); and "Kidney Stones
Frequently Asked Questions," Your Medical Source, http://yourmedicalsource
.com/library/kidneystones/KS_faq.html (accessed January 27, 2004).

27. The role of clotting in calcification is under investigation by a team led by
E. Olavi Kajander at Nanobac Life Sciences in Tampa, Florida. Interview by
the authors with Kajander, April 26, 2003.

28. This is the emerging theory of atherogenesis referred to later in the book.

29. The toxicity of hydroxyl apatite particles has been well known for many years.
"BCP crystals stimulate release of prostaglandins during endocytosis by
synovial cells lining the joint space. Within cells they cause relentless release
of neutral proteases and act as growth factors, stimulating cell division.
These properties have been linked with the destructive joint changes. When
BCP crystals rupture into a joint or in cases of calcific periarthritis, they
may attract neutrophils and cause an acute inflammation, which is often
severe." "Basic Calcium Phosphate and Other Crystal Disorders," *The Merck
Manual of Diagnosis and Therapy*, sec. 5. Musculoskeletal and Connective

Tissue Disorders, chap. 55, Crystal-Induced Conditions, http://www.merck
.com/mrkshared/mmanual/section5/chapter55/55d.jsp (accessed March 1,
2004). Also, "We found that basic calcium phosphate (BCP) crystals greatly
stimulated the endocytotic activity of cells by rendering the cells more
permeable and that the anti-calcification agent phosphocitrate and several
others inhibited the crystals-mediated endocytosis." Sun et al., "Basic Calcium
Phosphate Crystals Stimulate the Endocytotic Activity of Cells: Inhibition
by Anti-calcification Agents," *Biochem Biophys Res Commun* 312, no. 4
(December 2003): 1053–59. Despite these clear findings, the toxic effects of
calcium phosphate particles are usually downplayed in daily medicine, and
patients are unaware of the impacts.

30. Daniel Q. Haney, "Vulnerable Plaque: The Latest in Heart Disease?" *Associated Press*, January 11, 1999, http://www.canoe.com/Health9901/11_heart
.html (accessed April 25, 2004). "By the time you see an irregularity on the
angiogram, the first little 25 per cent narrowing, over 85 per cent of the
rest of the arteries are atherosclerotic. It's all hidden." Dr. Steven Nissen,
Cleveland Clinic.

31. "Coronary Artery Disease," *The Harvard Medical School Family Health Guide*
(New York: Simon and Schuster, 1999, updated 2003), http://www.health
.harvard.edu/fhg/fhgupdate/K/K2.shtml (accessed April 14, 2004).

32. "Toshiba Receives FDA Clearance on Cardiac Functional Analysis Package
for the Aquilion™16 Multislice CT Scanner, Tustin, California," December
18, 2002, http://www.medical.toshiba.com/news/pressreleases/121802-434
.htm (accessed April 17, 2004).

CHAPTER 3: THE NANOBACTERIA DETECTIVES

1. A description of how the polio vaccine is prepared is found in "The Withdrawal of an Oral Polio Vaccine: Analysis of Events and Implications; A
Report by the Chief Medical Officer CMO OPV," June 2002, Department of
Health, UK, http://www.publications.doh.gov.uk/cmo/opvreport/opvrepjun02
.pdf (accessed March 30, 2004).

2. Christine Stencel and Cory Arberg, "More Data Needed to Determine
If Contaminated Polio Vaccine from 1955–1963 Causes Cancer in Adults
Today," National Academies, Press Release, October 22, 2002, http://www4
.nas.edu/news.nsf/isbn/0309086108?OpenDocument (accessed January 18,
2004). New reports also suggest that contaminated vaccines from the Soviet
era may have been used in Eastern Europe and elsewhere after 1963. Debbie
Bookchin, "Vaccine Scandal Revives Cancer Fear," *New Scientist* 183, no.
2455 (July 10, 2004): 6.

3. In 2004, Professor Carson was director of the Sam and Rose Stein Institute
for Research on Aging at the University of California, San Diego.

4. Joel B. Baseman and Joseph G. Tully, "Mycoplasmas: Sophisticated,
Reemerging, and Burdened by Their Notoriety," *Emerging Infectious Diseases*
3, no.1 (January–March 1997): 21–32.

5. Interview by the authors with E. Olavi Kajander, April 23, 2003.

6. United States Patent Office, patent no. 5,135,851.

7. Interview by the authors with E. Olavi Kajander, October 15, 2002.

8. "Diagnosis of mycoplasma infections...has had a troubling history... With the application of molecular genetic technology, new methods have been developed such as DNA fingerprinting . . . " Quote from David MacKenzie, "Epidemiology and Control of Emerging Strains of Poultry Respiratory Disease Agents," Northeastern Regional Association of State Agricultural Experiment Station Directors, November 10, 2002, http://www.lgu.umd .edu/project/outline.cfm?trackID=10#top (accessed April 10, 2004).

9. J. Westberg, A. Persson, A. Holmberg, A. Goesmann, J. Lundeberg, K. E. Johansson, B. Pettersson, M. Uhlen, "The Genome Sequence of *Mycoplasma mycoides* subsp. mycoides SC Type Strain PG1T, the Causative Agent of Contagious Bovine Pleuropneumonia (CBPP)," *Genome Res* 14, no. 2 (February 2004): 221–27. Also, Syed A. Bokhari, "*Mycoplasma gallisepticum*," excerpt published by State of Colorado Department of Agriculture Web site, http://ag.state.co.us/animals/livestock_disease/mycopl.html (accessed August 15, 2004).

10. N. Çiftçioğlu and O. Kajander, "Growth Factors of Nanobacteria," *Proceedings SPIE,* vol. 3755: 113–19.

11. T. G. Harrison and N. Doshi, "Serological Evidence of *Bartonella spp.* Infection in the UK," *Epidemiol Infect* 123, no. 2 (October 1999): 233–40. Also, a general observation: Microbiologists have known for years that infections survive for long periods in the blood, but some medical Web sites and articles still claim, based on outdated concepts, that healthy blood is sterile.

12. "Basic Calcium Phosphate and Other Crystal Disorders," *The Merck Manual of Diagnosis and Therapy,* sec. 5, Musculoskeletal and Connective Tissue Disorders, chap. 55, Crystal-Induced Conditions, http://www.merck.com/mrkshared/mmanual/section5/chapter55/55d.jsp (accessed March 1, 2004).

13. Robert Kunzig, "The Unbearably Unstoppable Neutrino," *Discover Magazine* 22, no. 8 (August 2001): 40.

14. E. Olavi Kajander, Mikael Björklund, and Neva Çiftçioğlu, "Suggestions from Observations on Nanobacteria Isolated From Blood," Panel 2, Size Limits of Very Small Microorganisms, Proceedings of a Workshop, Washington, D.C., October 22–23, 1998, Space Studies Board, National Academy of Sciences, http://www7.nationalacademies.org/ssb/nanopanel2Kajander.html (accessed March 30, 2004).

15. N. Çiftçioğlu, M. A. Miller-Hjelle, J. T. Hjelle, and E. O. Kajander, "Inhibition of Nanobacteria by Antimicrobial Drugs As Measured by a Modified Microdilution Method," *Antimicrobial Agents and Chemotherapy* 46, no. 7 (July 2002): 2077–86, http://www.pubmedcentral.nih.gov/articlerender .fcgi?artid=127303 (accessed August 15, 2004).

CHAPTER 4: CHALLENGING THE DEFINITION OF LIFE

1. "Cold Fusion Farewell," *New Scientist* 157, no. 2126 (March 21, 1998): 23.

2. According to Jack Maniloff of the University of Rochester, "it is the cold fusion of microbiology." Jenny Hogan, "Are Nanobacteria Alive or Just Strange Crystals?" *New Scientist* 182, no. 2448 (May 22, 2004): 6.

3. L. G. Puskás, L. Tiszlavicz, L. Torday, J. Papp, "Detection of *Nanobacterium sanguineum* in Human Atherosclerotic Plaques," International Nanobacteria

Minisymposium, Kuopio, Finland, March 8, 2001, Book of Abstracts, Kuopio University Press, Kuopio (in press). Abstract published online at http://www .nanobac.com/nbminisymp080301 (accessed May 15, 2004).

4. Todd E. Rasmussen, Brenda L. Kirkland, Jon Charlesworth, George P. Rodgers, Sandra R. Severson, Jeri Rodgers, Robert L. Folk, and Virginia M. Miller, "Electron Microscope and Immunological Evidence of Nanobacterial-like Structures in Calcified Carotid Arteries, Aortic Aneurysms and Cardiac Valves," *J Am Coll Cardiol (JACC)* 39, no. 5 (March 6, 2002): Supplement A. Also, John C. Lieske, Vivek Kumar, Gerard Farell-Baril, Shihui Yu, Jon E. Charlesworth, Ewa Rzewuska-Lech, Peter LaBreche, Sandra R. Severson, and Virginia M. Miller, "Detection and Propagation of Calcified Nanostructures from Human Aneurysms," *JACC Abstract Book* 43, no. 5 (March 2004) 1059–13: p. 13A [presented at the American College of Cardiology Annual Scientific Session 2004 in New Orleans, LA, on March 8, 2004]. And, Virginia M. Miller, George Rodgers, Jon A. Charlesworth, Brenda Kirkland, Sandra R. Severson, Todd E. Rasmussen, Marineh Yagubyan, Jeri C. Rodgers, Franklin R. Cockerill, Robert L. Folk, Vivek Kumar, Gerard Farell-Baril and John C. Lieske, "Evidence of Nanobacterial-like Structures in Human Calcified Arteries and Cardiac Valves,"*Am J Physiol Heart Circ Physiol* 287, no. 3 (September 2004): H1115–24.

5. J. T. Hjelle, M. A. Miller-Hjelle, I. R. Poxton, O. Kajander, N. Çiftçioğlu, M. L. Jones, R. C. Caughey, R. Brown, P. D. Millikin, and F. S. Darras, "Endotoxin and Nanobacteria in Polycystic Kidney Disease," *Kidney International* 57 (2000): 2360–74.

6. M. Khullar, S. K. Sharma, S. K. Singh, P. Bajwa, F. A. Sheikh, V. Relan, and M. Sharma, "Morphological and Immunological Characteristics of Nanobacteria from Human Renal Stones of a North Indian Population," *Urol Res* 32, no. 3 (June 2004): 190–95.

7. R. Sedivy and W. B. Battistutti, "Nanobacteria Promote Crystallization of Psammoma Bodies in Ovarian Cancer," *APMIS* 111, no. 10 (October 2003): 951–54.

8. T. M. Jelic, A. M. Malas, S. S. Groves, B. Jin, P.F. Mellen, G. Osborne, R. Roque, J. G. Rosencrance, and H. H. Chang, "Nanobacteria-Caused Mitral Valve Calciphylaxis in a Man with Diabetic Renal Failure," *South Med J* 97, no. 2 (February 2004): 194–98.

9. Robert L. Folk, "Nanobacteria: Surely Not Figments, but What Under Heaven Are They?" *Natural Science* 1, article 3 (1997), http://naturalscience .com/ns/articles/01-03/ns_folk.html (accessed January 25, 2004).

10. The term "nannobacteria" (with two *n*'s) was first used in scientific literature by Richard Y. Morita, "Bioavailibility of Energy and Starvation Survival in Nature," *Canadian Journal of Microbiology* 34 (1988): 436–41. Also, Folk, "Nanobacteria: Surely Not Figments, but What Under Heaven Are They?"

11. D. S. McKay, E. K. Gibson Jr., K. L. Thomas-Keprta, H. Vali, C. S. Romanek, S. J. Clemett, X. D. F. Chillier, C. R. Maechling, R. N. Zare, "Search for Past Life on Mars: Possible Relic Biogenic Activity in Martian Meteorite ALH84001," *Science* 273, no. 5277 (August 16, 1996): 924–30.

12. N. Boyce, "The Martians in Your Kidneys," *New Scientist* 163, no. 2200 (August 21, 1999): 32.

Notes

13. Philippa J. R. Uwins, Richard I. Webb, and Anthony P. Taylor, "Novel Nano-Organisms from Australian Sandstone," *American Mineralogist* 83 (1998): 1541–50, http://www.microscopy-uk.org.uk/nanobes/nanobes.pdf (accessed January 20, 2004). See also Dr. Uwins's Web site at http://www.uq.edu.au/nanoworld/uwins.html (accessed January 20, 2004).

14. Ibid.

15. Harald Huber, Michael J. Hohn, Reinhard Rachel, Tanja Fuchs, Verena C. Wimmer, and Karl O. Stetter, "A New Phylum of Archaea Represented by a Nanosized Hyperthermophilic Symbiont," *Nature* 417 (May 2, 2002): 63–67, http://www.nature.com/cgi-taf/Dynapage.taf?file=/nature/journal/v417/n6884/abs/417063a_fs.html (accessed January 20, 2004).

16. Elizabeth Waters, Michael J. Hohn, Ivan Ahel, David E. Graham, Mark D. Adams, Mary Barnstead, Karen Y. Beeson, Lisa Bibbs, Randall Bolanos, Martin Keller, Keith Kretz, Xiaoying Lin, Eric Mathur, Jingwei Ni, Mircea Podar, Toby Richardson, Granger G. Sutton, Melvin Simon, Dieter Söll, Karl O. Stetter, Jay M. Short, and Michiel Noordewier, "The Genome of *Nanoarchaeum equitans*: Insights into Early Archaeal Evolution and Derived Parasitism," *PNAS* 100, no. 22 (October 28, 2003): 12984–88.

17. Carson, "An Infectious Origin of Extraskeletal Calcification," *Proceedings of the National Academy of Sciences* 95 (1998): 7846–47.

18. "We have enough evidence to suggest that these microparticles are living microorganisms." Khullar et al., "Morphological and Immunological Characteristics of Nanobacteria," *Urol Res* 32, no. 3 (June 2004): 190–95.

19. Jelic et al., "Nanobacteria-caused Mitral Valve Calciphylaxis," *South Med J* 97, no. 2 (February 2004): 194–98.

20. Interview by the authors with E. Olavi Kajander, October 15, 2002. Also, N. Çiftçioğlu, E. O. Kajander, "Interaction of Nanobacteria with Cultured Mammalian Cells," *Pathophysiology* 4 (1998): 259–70. The total definition is far more complex, as we see in the rest of this chapter.

21. Charles F. A. Bryce, "Alternative View on the Putative Organism, *Nanobacterium sanguineum*," Braids Education Consultants, Edinburgh EH10 6NZ, Scotland (undated), http://www.heartfixer.com/Nanobacterium-Report.htm (accessed January 23, 2004).

22. Sun et al., "Basic Calcium Phosphate Crystals Stimulate the Endocytotic Activity of Cells: Inhibition by Anti-calcification Agents," *Biochem Biophys Res Commun* 312, no. 4 (December 2003): 1053–59. Also, McCarthy et al., "Molecular Mechanism of Basic Calcium Phosphate Crystal-Induced Activation of Human Fibroblasts," *J Biol Chem* 273, no. 52 (December 25, 1998): 35161–69.

23. "Therefore, these nanostructures appear to synthesize RNA." Lieske et al., "Detection and Propagation of Calcified Nanostructures from Human Aneurysms," *JACC Abstract Book* 43, no. 5 (March 2004) 1059–13: p. 13A. "The presence of several distinct protein bands suggests that these bacteria have protein synthesizing machinery." Khullar et al., "Morphological and Immunological Characteristics of Nanobacteria," *Urol Res* 32, no. 3 (June 2004): 190–95.

24. Katja Aho and E. Olavi Kajander, "Pitfalls in the Detection of Novel Nano-organisms," Letters to the Editor, *Journal of Clinical Microbiology* 41, no. 7

(July 2003): 3460–61. This letter compares the characteristics of nanobacteria with other pathogens, such as viruses and conventionally known bacteria, presenting data that nanobacteria are a unique life form.

25. Kenneth Nealson, "Panel 2 Discussion Summarized by K. Nealson," Size Limits of Very Small Microorganisms, Proceedings of a Workshop, Washington, D.C., October 22–23, 1998, Space Studies Board, National Academy of Sciences, http://www7.nationalacademies.org/ssb/nanopanel2.html (accessed March 30, 2003). "A NASA Workshop on Size Limits of Very Small Microorganisms agreed that a minimal living nanobe would require enough DNA for a core set of 250 proteins and at least one ribosome. A ribosome is a structure possessed by all known life forms; it acts like a workbench where proteins are hammered out according to the specs contained in the DNA. No ribosome, no proteins. All the DNA in the world won't help if you can't translate it into working proteins. As far as size is concerned, the ribosome is the kicker. It's at least 25 nanometers wide, all by itself. If you wadded up the core DNA along with the required ribosome, the tightest ball you can get would be about 200 nanometers in diameter. This might explain the largest of the nanobacteria, but it seemed to rule out the smaller ones, some of which are smaller than the ribosome alone." Scott Anderson, "The Attack of the Killer Nanobacteria," Science for People (June 13, 2004), http://www.scienceforpeople.com (accessed June 15, 2004).

26. Kajander, Björklund, and Çiftçioğlu, "Suggestions from Observations on Nanobacteria Isolated from Blood," Panel 2, Size Limits of Very Small Microorganisms, Proceedings of a Workshop, Washington, D.C., October 22–23, 1998, Space Studies Board, National Academy of Sciences, http://www7.nationalacademies.org/ssb/nanopanel2Kajander.html (accessed March 30, 2004).

27. Interview by the authors with E. Olavi Kajander, October 16, 2002.

28. Note from Gary Mezo to the authors, May 5, 2003.

29. Jeffrey G. Lawrence, "Gene Transfer and Minimal Genome Size," Panel 1, Size Limits of Very Small Microorganisms, Proceedings of a Workshop, Washington, D.C., October 22–23, 1998, Space Studies Board, National Academy of Sciences, http://www7.nationalacademies.org/ssb/nanopanel1lawrence.html (accessed April 30, 2004).

30. E. Olavi Kajander, "Alleged Nanobacteria Exist and Participate in Calcification of Arterial Plaque, Response to November 2002 issue having Elmer M. Cranton's letter 'Alleged Nanobacteria Do Not Cause Calcification of Arterial Plaque,'" Nanobac Oy Web site, http://www.nanobac.com/Klin%20lab/press.htm (accessed January 20, 2004). See also discussion paper with that comparison: Peter B. Moore, "A Biophysical Chemist's Thoughts on Cell Size," Panel 1, Size Limits of Very Small Microorganisms, Proceedings of a Workshop, Washington, D.C., October 22–23, 1998, Space Studies Board, National Academy of Sciences, http://www7.nationalacademies.org/ssb/nanopanel1moore.html (accessed March 20, 2004).

31. Alison Abbott, "Battle Lines Drawn between 'Nanobacteria' Researchers," *Nature* 401 (September 9, 1999): 105.

32. E-mail from Matti Uusitupa Rector, University of Kuopio, Finland, to Douglas Mulhall, November 21, 2002.

33. According to Kajander, the complaint was later filed with the Central Science Ethics Committee of Finland (approx. translation of title), where it was also rejected. Interview by the authors with E. Olavi Kajander, April 23, 2003.

34. John O. Cisar, De-Qi Xu, John Thompson, William Swaim, Lan Hu, and Dennis J. Kopecko, "An Alternative Interpretation of Nanobacteria-Induced Biomineralization," *Proceedings of the National Academy of Sciences* 97 (October 10, 2000): 11511–15.

35. Open Session Minutes, Food and Drug Administration, Center for Biologics Evaluation and Research, Vaccines and Biological Products Advisory Committee, Bethesda Maryland, November 18, 2002, http://www.fda.gov/ohrms/dockets/ac/02/transcripts/3906T1.doc (accessed April 30, 2004). Note: Kajander's name was misspelled in the minutes as "Pejander."

36. E. Olavi Kajander, Neva Çiftçioğlu, and Katja M. Aho, "Detection of Nanobacteria in Viral Vaccines," *Proceedings of the American Society for Microbiology*, 101st General Meeting, Orlando, FL, May 20–24, 2001, http://www.asmusa.org/memonly/abstracts/AbstractView.asp?AbstractID= 50191 (accessed March 30, 2004).

37. Open Session Minutes, Food and Drug Administration, transcript, p. 14.

38. Cisar et al., "An Alternative Interpretation of Nanobacteria-Induced Biomineralization," *PNAS* 97 (October 10, 2000).

39. Correspondence from Dr. Kopecko to the authors, June 6, 2003.

40. Hogan, "Are Nanobacteria Alive or Just Strange Crystals?" *New Scientist* 182, no. 2448 (May 22, 2004): 6.

41. Open Session Minutes, Food and Drug Administration, transcript, p. 14.

42. Cisar et al., "An Alternative Interpretation of Nanobacteria-Induced Biomineralization." The FDA Web site, http://www.fda.gov/cber/research/0500707.htm (accessed August 15, 2004), also cites J. O. Cisar, D. Q. Xu, J. Thompson, W. Swaim, L. Hu, and D. J. Kopecko, "Absence of Nanobacteria in Human Saliva and Dental Plaque," *Dental Research* 79 (Special Issue 2000): 2231.

43. Kajander, "Alleged Nanobacteria Exist and Participate in Calcification of Arterial Plaque, Response to November 2002 issue having Elmer M. Cranton's letter 'Alleged Nanobacteria Do Not Cause Calcification of Arterial Plaque'," Nanobac Oy Web site, http://www.nanobac.com/Klin%20lab/press.htm (accessed January 20, 2004).

44. Ibid.

45. Correspondence from Dennis J. Kopecko to the authors, June 6, 2003, and from E. Olavi Kajander to the authors, June 19, 2003.

46. Correspondence from E. Olavi Kajander to the authors, June 19, 2003.

47. "[W]e have never noticed formation of biofilm on plastic surfaces." Michel Drancourt, Véronique Jacomo, Hubert Lépidi, Eric Lechevallier, Vincent Grisoni, Christian Coulange, Edith Ragni, Claude Alasia, Bertrand Dussol, Yvon Berland, and Didier Raoult, "Attempted Isolation of *Nanobacterium sp.* Microorganisms from Upper Urinary Tract Stones," *Journal of Clinical Microbiology* 41, no. 1 (January 2003): 368–72, abstract, http://jcm.asm.org/cgi/content/abstract/41/1/368 (accessed February 15, 2004).

48. Telephone interview by the authors with Neva Çiftçioğlu, January 15, 2003.

49. These allegations and rebuttals occurred in e-mail messages sent to the authors by a journalist from a technology magazine and from Kajander and Çiftçioğlu throughout May 2004.

50. Hogan, "Are Nanobacteria Alive or Just Strange Crystals?" *New Scientist.*

51. E. Olavi Kajander and Neva Çiftçioğlu, "Nanobacteria: An Alternative Mechanism for Pathogenic Intra- and Extracellular Calcification and Stone Formation," *Proceedings of the National Academy of Sciences (PNAS)* USA 95, no. 14 (1998): 8274–79.

52. A. P Sommer, U. Oron, A.-M. Pretorius, D. S. McKay, N. Çiftçioğlu, A. R. Mester, E. O. Kajander, and H. T. Whelan, "A Preliminary Investigation into Light Modulated Replication of Nanobacteria and Heart Disease," *Journal of Clinical Laser Medicine and Surgery* 21, no. 4 (August 1, 2003): 231–35.

53. E. Olavi Kajander, "Nanobacteria Are Not Just Apatite," slide 38 from PowerPoint presentation provided to the authors, March 2004.

54. Rasmussen et al., "Electron Microscopic and Immunological Evidence of Nanobacterial-Like Structures," *J Am Coll Cardiol* 39, no. 5 (March 6, 2002): Supplement A.

55. Puskás et al., "Detection of *Nanobacterium sanguineum* in Human Atherosclerotic Plaques," Int. Nanobacteria Minisymposium, Kuopio, Finland, March 8, 2001, Book of Abstracts, Kuopio University Press, Kuopio (in press).

56. Virginia M. Miller et al.,"Evidence of Nanobacterial-like Structures in Human Calcified Arteries and Cardiac Valves," *Am J Physiol Heart Circ Physiol* 287, no. 3 (September 2004): H1115–24.

57. "People who received polio vaccine between 1954 and 1962 may have received a dose that contained SV40. As many as 10 to 30 million persons in the U.S. could have received SV40-contaminated injectable polio vaccine." "Concerns about Vaccine Contamination," Centers for Disease Control Web site, http://www.cdc.gov/nip/vacsafe/concerns/gen/contamination.htm (accessed January 26, 2004).

58. "Kidney Stones in Adults," National Kidney and Urologic Disease Clearinghouse, National Institutes of Health, http://www.niddk.nih.gov/health/kidney/pubs/stonadul/stonadul.htm#who (accessed March 27, 2004).

59. Ibid.

60. Ibid.

61. "What Causes Kidney Stones?" UC Davis Health System Medical Conditions A–Z list 2001, http://www.ucdmc.ucdavis.edu/ucdhs/health/a-z/81kidneystones/doc81causes.html (accessed April 17, 2004).

62. Kajander and Çiftçioğlu, "Nanobacteria: An Alternative Mechanism for Pathogenic Intra- and Extracellular Calcification and Stone Formation," *Proceedings of the National Academy of Sciences (PNAS)* USA 95, no. 14 (1998): 8274–79.

63. Ibid.

64. "Learning about Polycystic Kidney Disease," The PKD Foundation, http://www.pkdcure.org/aboutPkd.htm (accessed March 29, 2004).

65. Hjelle et al., "Endotoxin and Nanobacteria in Polycystic Kidney Disease," *Kidney International* 57 (2000): 2360–74.

66. Ibid.

67. The study "Pathogenesis of Calcium Nephrolithiasis," directed by Fredric Coe, has been awarded financing by the NIH for fiscal years 1998–2002; see http://grants2.nih.gov/grants/award/state/fy2000.illinois.txt (accessed April 10, 2004). Also, NIH, PO 1 DK 56788, "Pathogenesis and Treatment of Calcium Nephrolithiasis," F. L. Coe, Principal Investigator; Project 3 - "Mechanism of Stone Formation in the Rat and Core C: Genetic Hypercalciuric Stone Form-ing Rats," D. A. Bushinsky, Principal Investigator, http://www.urmc.rochester .edu/MEDICINE/media/dynamic/application/pdf/EndoFac.pdf (accessed April 30, 2004). Coe emphasized in an e-mail message to the authors, June 23, 2003, that his research has nothing to do with research by the scientists who are working on nanobacteria. However, we have included reference to Coe's work here due to the apparent similarities between the calcium phosphate found in his new studies and the material found by nanobacterial researchers in kidney stones.

68. Andrew P. Evan, James E. Lingerman, Fredric L. Coe, Joan H. Parks, Sharon B. Bledsoe, Youzhi Shao, Andre J. Sommer, Ryan F. Paterson, Ramsay L. Kuo, and Marc Grynpas, "Randall's Plaque of Patients with Nephrolithiasis Begins in Basement Membranes of Thin Loops of Henle," *Journal of Clinical Investigation* 111 (2003): 607–16.

69. Mayo Clinic researcher John Lieske is studying nanobacteria in kidney stones, http://mayoresearch.mayo.edu/mayo/research/staff/lieske_jc.cfm (accessed August 15, 2004).

70. Khullar et al., "Morphological and Immunological Characteristics of Nano-bacteria," *Urol Res* 32, no. 3 (June 2004): 190–95.

71. The paper cited a 1998 publication that had been published when it was still uncertain what nanobacteria were. Kajander and Çiftçioğlu, "Nanobacteria: An Alternative Mechanism for Pathogenic Intra- and Extracellular Calcifica-tion and Stone Formation," *Proceedings of the National Academy of Sciences (PNAS)* USA 95, no. 14 (1998): 8274–79.

72. Hjelle et al., "Endotoxin and Nanobacteria in Polycystic Kidney Disease," *Kidney International* 57 (2000): 2360–74.

73. Aho and Kajander, "Pitfalls in the Detection of Novel Nanoorganisms," Letters to the Editor, *Journal of Clinical Microbiology* 41, no. 7 (July 2003): 3460–61. This letter compares the characteristics of nanobacteria with other pathogens, such as viruses and conventionally known bacteria, presenting data that nanobacteria are a unique life form. The table is partially excerpted in this book as "How to Tell *Nanobacterium sanguineum*" (see fig. 8).

74. "Just as physicists recognize light either as electromagnetic waves or as par-ticulate photons, depending on the context, so biologists can profitably regard viruses both as exceptionally simple microbes and as exceptionally complex chemicals." R. Dulbecco and H. S. Ginsberg, *Virology* (Hagerstown, MD: Harper and Row, 1980) (originally published as a section of *Microbiology*, 3rd ed., by Davis et al. [Hagerstown, MD: Harper and Row, 1980], p. 855), http://web.uct.ac.za/microbiology/tutorial/molechis.htm (accessed March 18, 2004).

CHAPTER 5: SEEDS OF DESTRUCTION

1. Rasmussen et al., "Electron Microscope and Immunological Evidence of Nanobacterial-like Structures," *J Am Coll Cardiol* 39, no. 5 (March 6, 2002): Supplement A.

2. Lieske et al., "Detection and Propagation of Calcified Nanostructures from Human Aneurysms," *JACC Abstract Book* 43, no. 5 (March 2004) 1059–13: p. 13A.

3. Jelic et al., "Nanobacteria-caused Mitral Valve Calciphylaxis in a Man with Diabetic Renal Failure," *South Med J* 97, no. 2 (February 2004): 194–98.

4. Lieske et al., "Detection and Propagation of Calcified Nanostructures from Human Aneurysms," *JACC Abstract Book*, 2004.

5. "Nanobac Life Sciences Announces Positive Results of its Nanobacterial Antibody Test for Coronary Artery Disease. Simple Blood Test Shows Correlation with Coronary Artery Calcification," Press Release, Nanobac Life Sciences, April 27, 2004, http://www.nanobaclabs.com/NewsRoom/PressReleases/Article.aspx?shortname=News_2004-04-27 (accessed April 27, 2004).

6. Benedict S. Maniscalco, "Shouldering the Risk Burden: Infection, Atherosclerosis, and the Vascular Endothelium," *Circulation* 107 (March 2003): 74. Also, Hyo-Chun Yoon, Aletha M. Emerick, Jennifer A. Hill, David W. Gjertson, and Jonathan G. Goldin, "Calcium Begets Calcium: Progression of Coronary Artery Calcification in Asymptomatic Subjects," *Radiology* 224 (2002): 236–41.

7. E. Olavi Kajander, M. Björklund, and N. Çiftçioğlu, "Nanobacteria and Man," in *Enigmatic Microorganisms and Life in Extreme Environments*, ed. J. Seckbach (Dordrecht, Netherlands: Kluwer Academic Publishers, 1999), 195–203. Also, interview between E. Olavi Kajander and the authors, April 22, 2003.

8. K. Ackerman, I. Kuronen, and O. Kajander, "Scanning Electron Microscopy of Nanobacteria—Novel Biofilm Producing Organisms in Blood," *Scanning* 15, no. III (1993).

9. "Identification of Bacterial Genes and Cell Structure(s) Inducing $CaCO_3$ Precipitation," Bioreinforce Project, EC Programme "Energy, Environment and Sustainable Development," http://www.ub.es/rpat/bioreinforce/ReportWeb .pdf (accessed April 17, 2004).

10. Kajander et al., "Nanobacteria and Man." Also, interview between the authors and E. Olavi Kajander, April 22, 2003.

11. E. Garcia-Cuerpo, E. O. Kajander, N. Çiftçioğlu, F. L. Castellano, C. Correa, J. Conzales, F. Mampaso, F. Liano, E. G. de Gabiola and Y. A. E. Berrilero, "Nanobacteria. Un Modelo de Neo-litogenesis Experimental," *Arch Esp Urol* 53, no. 4 (2000): 291–303. Also, E. Garcia-Cuerpo, E. O. Kajander, "Litogenesis. Hacia un nuevo planteamiento," *Arch Esp Urol* 54, no. 9 (2001): 851–53.

12. The role of nanobacteria in formation of kidney stones is summarized in E. Olavi Kajander, Neva Çiftçioğlu, Katja Aho, and Enrique Garcia-Cuerpo, "Characteristics of Nanobacteria and Their Possible Role in Stone Formation," Invited Editorial, *Urological Research* 31, no. 2 (June 2003): 47–54, abstract, http://link.springer.de/link/service/journals/00240/contents/03/00304/

Notes 199

(accessed April 30, 2004). For other research on formation of kidney stones due to calcification, see Evan et al., "Randall's Plaque of Patients with Neph-rolithiasis Begins in Basement Membranes of Thin Loops of Henle," *Journal of Clinical Investigation* 111 (2003): 607–16.

13. The discoveries of how nanobacteria act in atherosclerosis and how to get rid of them have a few turns to them. In 1998, the same year that Kajander and Çiftçioğlu applied to patent a treatment for nanobacteria infections, Professor Dennis Carson published his *PNAS* commentary "An Infectious Origin of Extraskeletal Calcification," *Proceedings of the National Academy of Sciences (PNAS)* that surmised, based on data from Kajander, Çiftçioğlu, and others, that nanobacteria and other pathogens may play a role in the body's inflammatory response to atherosclerotic vascular damage. Around 1999 László Puskás detected nanobacteria in atherosclerotic plaque. By then, the use of EDTA for dissolving calcium shells and the use of tetracycline for eliminating nanobacteria in vitro had been discovered and applied by Kajander and Çiftçioğlu since the early 1990s and published, for example, in "A New Potential Threat in Antigen and Antibody Products: Nanobacteria," Neva Çiftçioğlu, Ilpo Kuronen, Kari Akerman, Erkki Hiltunen, Jukka Laukkanen, and E. Olavi Kajander, in *Vaccines* 97, ed. F. Brown, D. Burton, P. Doharty, J. Mekalanos, and E. Norby (Cold Spring Harbor, NY: Cold Spring Harbor Laboratory Press, 1997). On the other hand, the discovery and practical work on how to effectively get rid of nanobacteria in atherosclerosis in vivo (i.e., in human subjects) was Gary Mezo's, based on Kajander and Çiftçioğlu's earlier EDTA and tetracycline combination. Mezo used other chemicals in a formula and sequence that made the combination work effectively in the human metabolism. This new combination succeeded, according to cardiologists interviewed for this book and the clinical trial supervised by Dr. Benedict Maniscalco, to measurably reverse the clinical signs of atherosclerosis in patients. Theorization about the pathophysiological role of nanobacteria has emerged from the confluence of those discoveries. Mezo maintained that he played the leading role in developing this "unifying theory of atherogenesis." Dr. Çiftçioğlu had a different view that, as with most theories, this one drew from earlier published works, in this case those done by Carson, Çiftçioğlu, Kajander, and others.

14. Sun et al., "Basic Calcium Phosphate Crystals Stimulate the Endocytotic Activity of Cells: Inhibition by Anti-calcification Agents," *Biochem Biophys Res Commun* 312, no. 4 (December 2003): 1053–59.

15. "Basic Calcium Phosphate and Other Crystal Disorders," *The Merck Manual of Diagnosis and Therapy*, sec. 5, Musculoskeletal and Connective Tissue Disorders, chap. 55, Crystal-Induced Conditions, http://www.merck.com/mrkshared/mmanual/section5/chapter55/55d.jsp (accessed March 1, 2004).

16. Sun et al., "Basic Calcium Phosphate Crystals Stimulate the Endocytotic Activity of Cells," *Biochem Biophys Res Commun* 312, no. 4 (December 2003): 1053–59.

17. Sedivy and Battistutti, "Nanobacteria Promote Crystallization of Psammoma Bodies in Ovarian Cancer," *APMIS* 111, no. 10 (October 2003): 951–54.

18. E. B. Breitschwerdt, Sushama Sontakke, Allen Cannedy, Susan I. Hancock, and Julie M. Bradley, "Infection with *Bartonella weissii* and Detection of Nanobacterium Antigens in a North Carolina Beef Herd," *Journal of Clinical Microbiology* 39 (2001): 879–82.

19. Philippe Brunet and Yvon Berland, "Water Quality Complications of Hae-
    modialysis," *Nephrology Dialysis Transplantation* 15 (2000): 578–80.

20. Neva Çiftçioğlu, "Screening of Human Gamma Globulin Products for
    Nanobacteria Markers," 102nd General Meeting of the American Society
    for Microbiology, Salt Lake City, UT, May 19–23, 2002 (Session 165, Pa-
    per Y-10), http://www.asmusa.org/memonly/abstracts/AbstractView.asp
    ?AbstractID=63965 (accessed March 30, 2004). For additional supporting
    data see next note.

21. Kajander, N. Çiftçioğlu, and Aho, "Detection of Nanobacteria in Viral
    Vaccines," *Proceedings of the American Society for Microbiology*, 101st
    General Meeting, Orlando, FL, May 20–24, 2001, http://www.asmusa.org/
    memonly/abstracts/AbstractView.asp?AbstractID=50191 (accessed March
    30, 2004). Also, M. Holmberg, "Prevalence of Human Anti-nanobacteria
    Antibodies Suggest Possible Zoonosis," abstract, International Nanobacteria
    Minisymposium, Kuopio, Finland, March 8, 2001, http://www.nanobac.com/
    nbminisymp080301/page10.html (accessed March 30, 2004).

Chapter 6: When to Declare "I'm Safe"

1. A check of many medical dictionaries, cancer Web sites, and infectious disease books will show variations on the technical definition of being "cured."
   The U.S. government's Medline Dictionary alone has varying definitions:
   "recovery from a disease <his *cure* was complete>; *also*: remission of signs or
   symptoms of a disease especially during a prolonged period of observation <a
   clinical *cure*> <5-year *cure* of cancer> . . . a course or period of treatment;
   especially: one designed to interrupt an addiction or compulsive habit or to improve general health . . ." Medline Medical Dictionary, U.S. National Library
   of Medicine, http://www2.merriam-webster.com/cgi-bin/mwmednlm?book=
   Medical&va=cure (accessed January 4, 2004).

2. Please refer to the note on definitions at the beginning of this book and the
   glossary for further explanation of the term "atherosclerosis."

3. "Coronary Artery Disease," *The Harvard Medical School Family Health Guide*
   (New York: Simon and Schuster, 1999, updated 2003), http://www.health
   .harvard.edu/fhg/fhgupdate/K/K2.shtml (accessed April 14, 2004).

4. Atherosclerosis has been the most pervasive cause of death worldwide compared to other diseases for some time. "Of more than 50 million deaths worldwide in 1997, about one-third were due to infectious and parasitic diseases
   such as acute lower respiratory diseases, tuberculosis, diarrhea, HIV/AIDS
   and malaria; about 30% were due to circulatory diseases such as coronary
   heart disease and cerebrovascular diseases [both are caused by atheroscle-
   rosis], and about 12% were due to cancers. While deaths due to circulatory
   diseases declined from 51% to 46% of total deaths in the developed world
   during the period 1985-1997, they increased from 16% to 24% of total deaths
   in the developing world." *The World Health Report 1998*, Executive Summary,
   World Health Organization, http://www.who.int/whr2001/2001/archives/1998/
   exsum98e.htm (accessed January 27, 2004).

5. David Satcher, "America Takes Heart Disease to Heart," Surgeon General,
   U.S. Department of Health and Human Services, January 24–28, 2000,
   http://www.health.gov/Partnerships/Media/heart.htm (accessed January 27,
   2004).

6. Mauri et al., "Comparison of Rotational Atherectomy with Conventional Balloon Angioplasty in the Prevention of Restenosis of Small Coronary Arteries: Results of the Dilatation vs Ablation Revascularization Trial Targeting Restenosis (DART)," *Am Heart J* 145, no. 5 (2003): 847–54, http://www.medscape.com/viewarticle/456231_print (accessed May 10, 2004). Also Winslow, "New Stents a Boon for Patients May Affect Rising Health Costs," *Wall Street Journal*, December 24, 2002, p. 1.

7. See the glossary for a definition of statins.

8. "A Cure for Cardiovascular Disease?" Editorial, *British Medical Journal* 326 (June 28, 2003): 1407–8.

9. Emma Ross, "Combination Pill Could Cut Heart Attacks and Strokes by About 80 Percent, Scientists Say," *Associated Press*, June 26, 2003.

10. Steven E. Nissen, Taro Tsunoda, E. Murat Tuzcu, Paul Schoenhagen, Christopher J. Cooper, Muhammad Yasin, Gregory M. Eaton, Michael A. Lauer, W. Scott Sheldon, Cindy L. Grines, Stephen Halpern, Tim Crowe, James C. Blankenship, and Richard Kerensky, "Effect of Recombinant ApoA-I Milano on Coronary Atherosclerosis in Patients with Acute Coronary Syndromes," *JAMA* 290, no. 17 (November 5, 2003): 2292–2300.

11. John McKenzie, "Reversing Heart Disease: Strain of Good Cholesterol Reduces Plaque in Coronary Arteries," ABC News.com, November 4, 2003, http://abcnews.go.com/sections/wnt/MedicineCuttingEdge/heartdisease_reverse031104.html (accessed February 10, 2004).

12. Nicholas Wade, "Company Ties Gene to Risk of Heart Attack and Stroke," *New York Times*, February 9, 2004, http://www.nytimes.com/2004/02/09/health/09GENE.html (accessed February 10, 2004).

13. Robert C. Atkins, *Dr. Atkins' New Diet Revolution* (New York: Avon Books, 1999, revised 2003). Various contradictory studies have been published on the effectiveness of the Atkins diet. By 2004, the Atkins "low carb" concept had evolved into a pervasive dietary fashion affecting everything from orange juice to meat and fast-food menus.

14. Arthur Agatston, *The South Beach Diet: The Delicious, Doctor-Designed, Foolproof Plan for Fast and Healthy Weight Loss* (New York: Rodale Press, 2003). The Agatston diet is similar in some ways to the Atkins diet. What makes it noteworthy is that Dr. Agatston is the pioneer of methods to measure calcium deposits in heart disease yet refrains in his book from claiming that his diet removes such deposits.

15. Dean Ornish, *Dr. Dean Ornish's Program for Reversing Heart Disease* (New York: Ballantine, 1992, revised 2003). Ornish has criticized the Atkins diet approach.

16. Matthias Rath, *Why Animals Don't Get Heart Attacks . . . But People Do!* (Fremont, CA: MR Publishing Inc, 2003). Rath is an outspoken proponent of using vitamins to promote cellular health.

17. Nobel laureate Linus Pauling's theory of heart disease claims that high doses of substances called lipoprotein(a) binding inhibitors prevent and dissolve the atherosclerotic plaques of heart disease. M. Rath and L. Pauling, "Solution of the Puzzle of Human Cardiovascular Disease: Its Primary Cause Is Ascorbate Deficiency, Leading to the Deposition of Lipoprotein(a) and

Fibrinogen/Fibrin in the Vascular Wall," *Journal of Orthomolecular Med* 6 (1991): 125–34.

18. "Unfortunately, the information embodied in this pyramid doesn't point the way to healthy eating. Why not? Its blueprint was based on shaky scientific evidence." "Food Pyramids. What Should You Really Eat?" Harvard School of Public Health, http://www.hsph.harvard.edu/nutritionsource/pyramids.html (accessed May 10, 2004).

19. "Questions and Answers: The NIH Trial of EDTA Chelation Therapy for Coronary Artery Disease," National Center for Complementary Medicine (August 7, 2002), http://nccam.nih.gov/news/2002/chelation/q-and-a.htm (accessed March 30, 2004).

20. One example relating to calcification is citrate, which is synthesized by the human metabolism and may be bolstered by diet.

21. The history of disinfection shows how long it has taken to put some medical discoveries into practice. Roman-era physicians sometimes sterilized their instruments for surgery and observed that this aided the healing process. Yet it was not until more than a millennium later that this knowledge was revived and advanced. Around 1500, Italian physician Girolamo Fracastoro theorized that invisible organisms cause disease. Then, another delay. It took until the 1850s for researchers such as Ignaz Semelweis, John Snow, and Heinrich Anton deBary to begin demonstrating the link between bacteria and disease. In 1867 Joseph Lister published the first work on antiseptic surgery, launching the trend toward aseptic techniques in medicine. Lansing M. Prescott, Donald A. Klein, and John P. Harley, *Microbiology*, McGraw Hill Learning Center, 2002, http://highered.mcgraw-hill.com/sites/0072320419/student_view0/interactive_time_line.html (accessed April 2, 2004).

22. Louis A. Dvonch and Russell Dvonch, *The Heart Attack Germ* (Lincoln, NE: I-universe, 2003).

23. A. Raza-Ahmad, G. A. Klassen, D. A. Murphy, J. A. Sullivan, C. E. Kinley, R. W. Landymore, and J. R. Wood, "Evidence of Type 2 Herpes Simplex Infection in Human Coronary Arteries at the Time of Coronary Artery Bypass Surgery," *Canadian Journal of Cardiology* 11, no. 11 (December 1995): 1025–29, http://www.pulsus.com/CARDIOL/11_11/Raza_ed.htm (accessed April 3, 2004).

24. This table draws from information provided in K. Bachmaier, J. Le, and J. M. Penninger, "Catching Heart Disease: Antigenic Mimicry and Bacterial Infections," *Nature Medicine* 6 (2000): 841–42. See also Aristo Vojdani, "A Look at Infectious Agents as a Possible Causative Factor in Cardiovascular Disease," *Laboratory Medicine* 34, no. 4 and 5 (April/May 2003).

25. Joseph Hodgson, *A Treatise on the Diseases of Arteries and Veins, Containing the Pathology and Treatment of Aneurysms and Wounded Arteries* (London: Printed by J. Moyes for Thomas Underwood, 1815). About a century and a half later, in 1976, Russell Ross theorized that heart disease was an inflammatory response to injury from disease. This work was updated in: R. Ross, "Mechanisms of Disease: Atherosclerosis—An Inflammatory Disease," [Review Article], *New England Journal of Medicine* 340 (1999): 115-26.

26. One example: Dvonch and Dvonch, *The Heart Attack Germ* (Lincoln, NE: I-universe, 2003). This book rightly identifies the signs of infection that have

been emerging in heart disease but then claims that there is proof to show the role of *Chlamydia pneumoniae* and other germs as the cause. Questions that remain unanswered are, are such germs involved at the beginning and do they trigger heart disease or just make it worse?

27. "Population studies have indicated a 1.5 to 2.0 times greater risk of fatal cardiovascular disease in patients with periodontal disease. In study after study, a positive connection has been found between oral disease and cardiovascular health." From "Oral Disease and Systemic Health: What Is the Connection?" American Association of Endodontists, http://www.aae.org/ss00ecfe.html (accessed April 4, 2004).

28. Christopher M. O'Connor, Michael W. Dunne, Marc A. Pfeffer, Joseph B. Muhlestein, Louis Yao, Sandeep Gupta, Rebecca J. Benner, Marian R. Fisher, Thomas D. Cook, "Azithromycin for the Secondary Prevention of Coronary Heart Disease Events," *Journal of the American Medical Association (JAMA)* 290, no. 11 (September 2003): 1459–66.

29. "Inflammation, Heart Disease and Stroke: The Role of C-Reactive Protein," American Heart Association, http://www.americanheart.org/presenter .jhtml?identifier=4648 (accessed April 3, 2004).

30. Ibid.

31. The story of *Helicobacter pylori* and the reluctance of medical authorities to acknowledge it as a cause of ulcers is well documented in many books and summarized in Ewald, *Plague Time: How Stealth Infections Cause Cancers, Heart Disease and Other Deadly Ailments* (New York: Anchor Books, 2002).

32. "*Helicobacter pylori* in Peptic Ulcer Disease," *NIH Consensus Statement Online 1994* 12, no. 1 (February 7–9, 1994): 1–23, http://consensus.nih.gov/ cons/094/094_statement.htm (accessed January 23, 2004).

33. Ibid.

34. "After the NIH recommendations were published, national surveys of primary care physicians and gastroenterologists indicated that approximately 90% of these physicians correctly identified *H. pylori* infection as the primary cause of ulcers. However, primary care physicians still reported treating more than 50% of their first time ulcer patients with acid-reducing medications and not antibiotic-based regimens." Benjamin D. Gold, "*H. pylori*: The Key to Cure for Most Ulcer Patients," http://www.cdc.gov/ulcer/keytocure.htm (accessed February 10, 2004).

35. Hemant Singhal, "Wound Infection," http://www.emedicine.com/med/ topic2422.htm (accessed January 5, 2004).

36. Alexander Fleming is credited with discovering penicillin in 1928 but only after many approaches had been tried by other researchers. Some methods such as sterilization had shown earlier but limited success. It took other scientists such as Howard Florey to find ways of mass manufacturing the drug many years later before it could come into broad use in World War II.

37. There is a rough historical parallel between the pathogens. Nanobacteria were discovered in 1985, shortly after *H. pylori* was found and treated in ulcers. However, it took much more time, until the late 1990s, for nanobacteria to be isolated in heart disease. News of that was published only in 2002. A way of eradicating nanobacteria had been known since the mid-1990s.

38. Paul Khairy, Stephane Rinfret, Jean-Claude Tardif, Richard Marchand, Stan Shapiro, James Brophy, Jocelyn Dupuis, "Absence of Association between Infectious Agents and Endothelial Function in Healthy Young Men," *Circulation* 107 (2003): 1966–71.

39. C. Espinola-Klein, H. J. Rupprecht, S. Blankenberg, C. Bickel, H. Kopp, A. Victor, G. Hafner, W. Prellwitz, W. Schlumberger, and J. Meyer, "Impact of Infectious Burden on Progression of Carotid Atherosclerosis," *Stroke* 33, no. 11 (November 2002): 2581–86.

40. Harvey McConnel, "Current Antibiotic Trials Test Role of Bacteria in Atherosclerosis," Doctor's Guide, August 1, 2002, http://www.docguide.com/news/content.nsf/news/8525697700573E1885256b51006ce88f?OpenDocument&id=48DDE4A73E09A9698526880078C249&c=Bacterial%20Infections&count=10 (accessed April 17, 2004), reviewing Maija Leinonen and Pekka Saikku, "Evidence for Infectious Agents in Cardiovascular Disease and Atherosclerosis," *Lancet Infectious Diseases* 2 (2002): 11–17. However, later studies suggest that while there may be short-term benefits from treating infections in heart disease with antibiotics, midterm impacts are negligable. O'Connor et al., "Azithromycin for the Secondary Prevention of Coronary Heart Disease Events."

41. Wade, "Company Ties Gene to Risk of Heart Attack and Stroke," *New York Times,* February 9, 2004, http://www.nytimes.com/2004/02/09/health/09GENE.html (accessed February 10, 2004).

CHAPTER 7: HOW DO I KNOW IF I HAVE THEM?

1. "Unfortunately, there is no clinically useful definitive assay for BCP crystals." "Basic Calcium Phosphate and Other Crystal Disorders," *The Merck Manual of Diagnosis and Therapy*, sec. 5, Musculoskeletal and Connective Tissue Disorders, chap. 55, Crystal-Induced Conditions, http://www.merck.com/mrkshared/mmanual/section5/chapter55/55d.jsp (accessed March 1, 2004).

2. "Nanobac Life Sciences Announces Positive Results of its Nanobacterial Antibody Test for Coronary Artery Disease. Simple Blood Test Shows Correlation with Coronary Artery Calcification," Press Release, Nanobac Life Sciences, April 27, 2004, http://www.nanobaclabs.com/NewsRoom/PressReleases/Article.aspx?shortname=News_2004-04-27 (accessed April 27, 2004).

3. The NanobacTEST U/A rapid ELISA test is an inexpensive on-the-spot urine test that checks for the presence of nanobacteria. The NanobacTEST-S is a serum blood test that checks for both nanobacterial antigen and antibodies in the blood. The original tests for detecting nanobacteria were developed by Drs. Kajander and Çiftçioğlu, then licensed to Nanobac Oy in Finland, which was subsequently acquired by Nanobac Life Sciences (formerly Nanobac Pharmaceuticals and NanobacLabs) in Tampa, Florida.

4. Holmberg, "Prevalence of Human Anti-Nanobacteria Antibodies Suggest Possible Zoonosis," abstract, International Nanobacteria Minisymposium, Kuopio, Finland, March 8, 2001, http://www.nanobac.com/nbminisymp080301/page10.html (accessed April 10, 2004).

5. According to E. Olavi Kajander and Benedict S. Maniscalco, 100 percent of their respective heart disease patients who were tested for nanobacteria

had positive results. Kajander maintains that "if you find nanobacteria in 15 percent of the general population (as a Finnish study did), then find that close to 100 percent of heart disease patients test positive, then that is significant." Interviews with Gary Mezo and E. Olavi Kajander, April 25, 2003, and with Benedict Maniscalco, March 16, 2003.

6. "CAT Scan," Medline Plus, National Institutes of Health, http://www.nlm .nih.gov/medlineplus/ency/article/003330.htm (accessed March 30, 2004).

7. The Nobel Prize in Physiology or Medicine for 1979 went jointly to Allan M. Cormack and Godfrey Newbold Hounsfield for the "development of computer assisted tomography." Press Release: "The 1979 Nobel Prize in Physiology or Medicine," http://www.nobel.se/medicine/laureates/1979/press.html (accessed May 10, 2004).

8. "Thoracic CT," Medline Plus, National Institutes of Health, http://www.nlm .nih.gov/medlineplus/ency/article/003788.htm (accessed January 21, 2004).

9. "Calcium Scan Predicts Heart Attack Risk in Physically Fit People," American Heart Association News Release, January 3, 2001, http://www.americanheart .org/presenter.jhtml?identifier=3292 (accessed April 3, 2004).

CHAPTER 8: CALCIUM GERM EXTERMINATORS

1. "Citrate is normal chelator (binder) of calcium, and low citrate levels in the urine may predispose to kidney calcification. Treatment with oral citrate has been used for over 3 years with no loss of metabolic control allowing normal-ization of urine citrate concentrations." David Weinstein, "Type I Glycogen Storage Disease: A Clinical and Research Update," Association for Glycogen Storage Disease, 2002 Workshop Report, http://www.agsd.org.uk/home/wrf .asp?F=2002_Workshop_Report.shtm (accessed April 25, 2004).

2. Dong Park Ki, Kyu Lee Won, Young Yun Ju, Keun Han Dong, Hyun Kim Soo, Ha Kim Young, Mook Kim Hyoung, and Taek Kim Kwang, "Novel Anti-calcification Treatment of Biological Tissues by Grafting of Sulphonated Poly(ethylene oxide)," *Biomaterials* 18, no. 1 (1997): 47–51.

3. Murray Epstein and Henry R. Black, "Arterial Calcification and Calcium Antagonists: What Does It Mean?" *Hypertension* 37 (2001): 1414, http://hyper .ahajournals.org/cgi/content/full/37/6/1414 (accessed April 25, 2004).

4. "Methods for Eradication of Nanobacteria," United States Patent Office, patent no. 6,706,290, published March 16, 2004, http://patft.uspto.gov/ netacgi/nph-Parser?Sect1=PTO1&Sect2=HITOFF&d=PALL&p=1&u=/ netahtml/srchnum.htm&r=1&f=G&l=50&s1=6706290.WKU.&OS=PN/ 6706290&RS=PN/6706290 (accessed March 25, 2004).

5. E. Olavi Kajander, "General Characteristics of Nanobacteria," slide 11, PowerPoint presentation, March 2004.

6. Jennifer Thomas, "Is There a Doctor in the House?" *HealthScout News*, Healthfinder, http://kcra-tvhealth.ip2m.com/index.cfm?PageType=itemDe tail&Item_ID=61955&Site_Cat_ID=15 (accessed March 3, 2004).

7. "Nutraceuticals (often referred to as phytochemicals or functional foods) are natural, bioactive chemical compounds that have health promoting, disease preventing or medicinal properties." The Nutraceutical Institute, http://foodsci.rutgers.edu/nci/#what (accessed January 21, 2004).

8. Whole books have been written about chelation. There is evidence on both sides about the success of the various types of chelation. Many patients and doctors swear by it. Other physicians say that it is dangerous. While we generally explain the role of EDTA as a sequestering agent for the purposes of describing the nanobiotic therapies, we as authors do not consider ourselves qualified to have a position on what is commonly referred to as "chelation." For that reason we have mentioned both sides of the discussion without comment. We also await the outcome of the National Institutes of Health study on this topic.

9. EDTA has been used for decades, sometimes with measurable results, other times with disputed ones. Its lead-removing properties have been known for many years. It has been the treatment of choice for heavy metal toxicity. D. O. Shiels, D. L. G. Thomas, and E. Kearley, "Treatment of Lead Poisoning by Edathamil Calcium-Disodium," *AMA Arch Indust Health* 13 (1956), 489, 497. It has been a generic medicine since the 1970s and is rated by the FDA as GRAS (generally recognized as safe). For a summary of other applications of EDTA, see "Questions and Answers: The NIH Trial of EDTA Chelation Therapy for Coronary Artery Disease," National Center for Complementary Medicine, August 7, 2002, http://nccam.nih.gov/news/2002/chelation/q-and-a.htm (accessed March 30, 2004).

10. Marsha Cohen, "Pharmacy Compounding," excerpted from chap. VIII, "Preparation of Drugs by a Pharmacy," *Pharmacy Law for California Pharmacists*, 4th ed., by William L. Marcus and Marsha N. Cohen (2002), http://www.uchastings.edu/cohen/gmos.htm (accessed March 30, 2004).

11. There are conflicting reports on chelation and kidney damage. A 2003 study found that EDTA chelation therapy may actually improve kidney function in some cases. See J.-L. Lin, D.-T. Lin-Tan, K.-H. Hsu, C.-C Yu, "Environmental Lead Exposure and Progression of Chronic Renal Diseases in Patients without Diabetes," *New England Journal of Medicine* 348 (January 23, 2003): 277–86. However, the American Cancer Society and other authorities say that chelation has the "potential" to cause kidney damage, although documentation on this claim is disputed. "Chelation," American Cancer Society Guide to Complementary and Alternative Methods, http://www.cancer.org/docroot/ETO/content/ETO_5_3X_Chelation_Therapy.asp?sitearea=ETO (accessed April 10, 2004).

12. In a note to the authors, May 5, 2003, Mezo indicated that he measured creatinine (a waste product from the body's use of protein) and BUN (blood urea nitrogen from the breakdown of blood, muscle, and protein). He also says he conducted liver function studies on patients.

13. Note from Gary Mezo to the authors, May 5, 2003.

14. E-mail communication from Katja M. Aho to the authors, March 9, 2004.

CHAPTER 9: REVERSING A SLOW-MOTION BLAST

1. Nanobac Life Sciences (previously Nanobac Pharmaceuticals and NanobacLabs) is the first company to commercialize nanobiotic treatments. The company has the most clinical experience and counts among its research collaborators E. Olavi Kajander, the discoverer who patented *Nanobacterium sanguineum*, and Dr. Neva Çiftçioğlu, the codeveloper of tests for detecting

it. It is the sole licensee of the original tests developed by Nanobac Oy in Finland for detecting such nanobacteria. In June 2003, American Enterprise Corporation acquired controlling interest in NanobacLabs through a share swap. The company then adopted the name Nanobac Pharmaceuticals, which was then superseded by Nanobac Life Sciences in April 2004. The information presented here about the treatment is gleaned from published research papers, the company's literature, and interviews with Dr. Kajander, Dr. Çiftçioğlu, Gary Mezo, and participating physicians as well as critics.

2. Most of the ingredients of the nutraceutical are described in the glossary.

3. "FDA has approved EDTA as a food additive that is generally recognized as safe (See the US Code of Federal Regulations-21 CFR 172.135 and 21 CFR 173.315)." "EDTA (ethylenediaminetetraacetic acid)," Whole Foods Health Information, http://www.wholefoods.com/healthinfo/edta.html (accessed March 15, 2004).

4. Ibid.

5. "Questions and Answers: The NIH Trial of EDTA Chelation Therapy for Coronary Artery Disease," National Center for Complementary Medicine (August 7, 2002), http://nccam.nih.gov/news/2002/chelation/q-and-a.htm (accessed March 30, 2004).

6. D. O. Shiels, D. L. G. Thomas, and E. Kearley, "Treatment of Lead Poisoning by Edathamil Calcium-Disodium," *AMA Arch Indust Health* 13 (1956), 489, 497. Also, "Questions and Answers: The NIH Trial of EDTA Chelation Therapy for Coronary Artery Disease."

7. Cardiologist James C. Roberts of Toledo, Ohio, who in the past has tried chelation therapy and vitamin therapy with patients, summarizes this view in a message to the authors, stating, "we know that IV and vitamin C confers tremendous benefits; just 1000 mg a day of vitamin C decreases 10-year event rate by 43 percent." Fax to the authors, April 2, 2003.

8. E. Cranton, A. Brecher, and J. Frackleton, *Bypassing Bypass: A Non-Surgical Therapy for Improving Circulation and Slowing the Aging Process* (Hampton Roads, VA: Medex Inc., 1980).

9. April Quinones, "EDTA Chelation and Calcium," http://www.anitafinley .com/sept00/calcium.html; see also "Magnesium EDTA, Chelation for Life," 2002, http://www.chelationforlife.com/Faqs/magnesium2.html (accessed March 31, 2004).

10. Todd J. Anderson, Jaroslav Hubacek, D. George Wyse, and Merril L. Knudtson, "Effect of Chelation Therapy on Endothelial Function in Patients with Coronary Artery Disease: PATCH Substudy," *J Am Coll Cardiol (JACC)* 41, no. 3 (February 5, 2003): 420–25. This study basically says that chelation therapy has no measurable positive impacts on patients with heart disease.

11. Ibid. Chelation therapists have vociferously rebutted the study. See Elmer Cranton, "Dr. Cranton's Rebuttal of the JAMA Article on IV Chelation Therapy," Chelation Therapy, http://www.chelationtherapyonline.com/ articles/p209.htm (accessed April 15, 2004).

12. Saul Green and Wallace Sampson, "EDTA Chelation Therapy for Atherosclerosis and Degenerative Diseases: Implausibility and Paradoxical Oxidant Effects," http://www.quackwatch.org/01QuackeryRelatedTopics/chelationimp .html (accessed March 30, 2004). This article cites as a basis for its claim about

skeptical medical associations "Diagnostic and Therapeutic Technology Assessment: Chelation Therapy," *JAMA* 250, no. 5 (1983): 672.

13. "Questions and Answers: The NIH Trial of EDTA Chelation Therapy for Coronary Artery Disease."

14. Ibid.

15. Interview with Gary Mezo, Tampa, Florida, October 16, 2002. The arguments presented in the ensuing paragraphs were made by Mezo based on his own experience and results obtained by physicians who participated in initial treatments of patients using nanobiotics. Mezo's position seems to have been at least partially supported by results from a clinical trial study of nanobiotics as described in chapter 10. However, that trial did not compare intravenous chelation with suppository-administered chelation. Nor did it compare use of the nutraceutical component with nonnutraceutical-enhanced chelation.

16. Interviews by the authors in late 2002 and early 2003 with James C. Roberts and other physicians who prescribe the nanobiotic therapy.

17. Correspondence from James C. Roberts to the authors, April 2, 2003.

18. Shiels et al., "Treatment of Lead Poisoning by Edathamil Calcium-Disodium." Also, "Questions and Answers: The NIH Trial of EDTA Chelation Therapy for Coronary Artery Disease."

19. "Method of Administering EDTA Complexes," United States Patent Office, patent no. 5,602,180, published February 11, 1997.

20. Interviews with Neva Çiftçioglu and E. Olavi Kajander, October 2002 through February 2003, based on their unpublished investigations.

21. N. Çiftçioglu et al., "Inhibition of Nanobacteria by Antimicrobial Drugs as Measured by a Modified Microdilution Method," *Antimicrobial Agents and Chemotherapy* 46, no. 7 (July 2002): 2077–86, http://www.pubmedcentral.nih .gov/articlerender.fcgi?artid=127303 (accessed August 15, 2004).

22. Harold W. Clark, "The Role of Chelation Therapy: Antibiotics and Mycoplasms," Portions taken from Harold W. Clark, "Why Arthritis? Searching for the Cause and the Cure of Rheumatoid Disease," http://www.arthritistrust .org/downloads/publications/pub115.pdf (accessed March 10, 2004).

23. "Fighting Arterial Plaque," Nanobac Sciences Inc. Web site, http://www .nanobacsciences.com/arterial_plaque.asp (accessed August 23, 2004).

24. Ibid.

25. "Noncompliance results in an estimated 125,000 deaths a year from cardiovascular disease alone, up to a quarter of nursing home admissions and an estimated 10% of hospital admissions." Delia O'Hara, "Given but Not Taken: When Your Patients Don't Take Their Medicines," American Medical News, February 4, 2002, http://www.ama-assn.org/amednews/2002/02/04/hlsa0204 .htm (accessed March 31, 2003).

CHAPTER 10: WHAT DOCTORS AND PATIENTS DISCOVERED

1. R. G. H., letter to NanobacLabs, February 11, 2002.

2. Excerpts from handwritten testimonials sent to NanobacLabs January to March, 2003.

3. Interview with Dr. C., April 10, 2003.

4. James C. Roberts Jr., "Overview," heartfixer.com, http://www.heartfixer .com/overview.htm (accessed April 29, 2004).

5. Correspondence from Dr. James C. Roberts to the authors, April 2, 2003.

6. James C. Roberts Jr., "*Nanobacterium sanguineum* Home Page," heartfixer .com, http://www.heartfixer.com/indexNB.htm (accessed April 29, 2004). Roberts has cited NanobacLabs's first in-house study of the impacts of NanobacTX on heart disease patients.

7. On the http://www.heartfixer.com Web site, there is a subsection entitled "*Nanobacterium sanguineum.*"

8. http://www.heartfixer.com/NB - Case Studies.htm (accessed April 15, 2004).

9. James C. Roberts Jr., "# 2 MP: NanobacTX for Atherosclerosis Everywhere," Patient Case Study, http://www.heartfixer.com/NB%20-%20Case%20Studies .htm##1-MP:%20%20NanobacTX%20for%20atherosclerosis%20everywh ere (accessed March 30, 2004).

10. http://www.heartfixer.com/NB - Case Studies.htm (accessed April 15, 2004).

11. Ibid.

12. Ibid.

13. Ibid.

14. Correspondence from Dr. James C. Roberts Jr. to the authors, April 2, 2003.

15. James C. Roberts Jr., "#15 MJ: The Up-Down Phenomena," Patient Case Study, http://www.heartfixer.com/NB%20-%20Case%20Studies.htm##15- MJ:%20%20The%20Up-Down%20Phenomena (accessed March 30, 2004).

16. Interview by the authors with Dr. Maniscalco, Tampa, Florida, October 16, 2002.

17. Ibid.

18. In 1997 at least 44,000 patients died from medical errors in the United States according to Linda T. Kohn, Janet M. Corrigan, Molla S. Donaldson, ed., *To Err Is Human: Building a Safer Health System, Institute of Medicine* (Washington, D.C.: National Academy Press, 1999). This data has been disputed, but its authoritative source suggests that medical error, especially in prescribing drugs is a problem. Newer Canadian studies also report many deaths from medical error. G. Ross Baker and Peter Norton, "Patient Safety and Healthcare Error in the Canadian Healthcare System, A Systematic Review and Analysis of Leading Practices in Canada with Reference to Key Initiatives Elsewhere," Health Canada, 2004, http://www.hc-sc.gc.ca/english/care/report/index.html (accessed August 20, 2004).

19. In "Why We're Losing the War on Cancer (and How to Win It)," the failure of the medical research establishment to find effective treatments for so many cancers is laid bare. Among the main criticisms: too much emphasis on costly clinical trials, combined with insufficient support for prevention and innovative ideas. Clifton Leaf, "Why We're Losing the War on Cancer (and How to Win It)," *Fortune* 149, no. 6 (March 22, 2004): 76–97.

20. D. M. Eisenberg, R. B. Davis, S. Ettner, S. Appel, S. Wilkey, M. Van Rompay, and R. C. Kessler, "Trends in Alternative Medicine Use in the United States 1990–97: Results of a Follow-up National Survey," *JAMA* 280 (1998): 1569–75.

21. Nancy Keates, "The Holistic Hospital," *Wall Street Journal,* March 28, 2003, W1.

22. Tinker Ready, "Trials Suspended Due to Death at Hopkins," *Nature Medicine* 7, no. 8 (August 2001): 877.

23. The Western IRB is not a testing agency but rather sets the ground rules for studies on new treatments. Its mission is to "Protect the Rights and Welfare of the Human Research Subject." It is the oldest and most experienced independent IRB in America. The board has reviewed research by more than 10,000 investigators in over thirty countries, and in every U.S. state. Western IRB Web site, http://www.wirb.com/ (accessed January 21, 2004).

24. Interview with Dr. Maniscalco, October 16, 2002.

25. Ibid.

26. Ibid.

27. The clinical trial study results that Maniscalco cites have been accepted for publishing as B. S. Maniscalco and K. A. Taylor, "Calcification in Coronary Artery Disease Can Be Reversed by EDTA–Tetracycline Long-Term Chemotherapy," *Pathophysiology* DOI:10.1016/j.pathophys.2004.06.001 (accepted June 3, 2004). Other comments in this section are taken from interviews with Dr. Maniscalco, October 16, 2002, and March 19, 2003.

28. Interview with Dr. Maniscalco, October 16, 2002.

29. Ibid.

30. Interview with J. K., October 31, 2002.

31. Interview with Dr. C., April 10, 2003.

32. Interviews with E. Olavi Kajander and Neva Çiftçioğlu, January–March 2004. Not much is published on this structural difference, but it can be seen in electron microscope photographs of bone matrix versus the shell structure of nanobacteria.

CHAPTER 11: CAN WE ALL BE PROTECTED?

1. This quote from Dr. Roberts's Web site was modified as a result of correspondence with Dr. Roberts, April 2, 2003. See http://www.heartfixer.com for more information. Dr. Roberts has used NanobacTX in combination with enhanced external counter pulsation (EECP), a therapy to help the body naturally bypass blocked arteries.

2. Rauno Harvima, "Association of Nanobacteria with Dermatological Diseases," Nanobac Life Sciences Web site, http://www.nanobaclabs.com/Research/Abstracts/PopUp.aspx?shortname=abstract10 (accessed August 15, 2004).

3. "The Jarisch-Herxheimer reaction describes the release of endotoxin when large numbers of organisms are killed by antibiotics." Jarisch-Herxheimer reaction, General Practice Notebook—a UK medical encyclopedia on the

World Wide Web, http://www.gpnotebook.co.uk/cache/2140798985.htm (accessed April 15, 2004).

4. M. Y. Rabau, M. Baratz, P. Rozen, "Na2 Ethylenediamine-tetraacetic Acid Retention Enema in Dogs: Biochemical and Histological Response," *General Pharmacology* 22, no. 2 (1991): 329–30.

5. Interviews by the authors with Drs. Maniscalco, Roberts, and other physicians between October 2002 and May 2003.

6. A NanobacTX ACES Clinical Study carried out by NanobacLabs (now Nanobac Life Sciences) showed decreases in coronary artery calcification, with EBCT scores reduced by an average of 58 percent, according to Kajander et al., "The Pathogenesis of Vascular Calcification," Poster session, Tampere, Finland, February 21, 2003. Dr. James C. Roberts and Dr. Benedict Maniscalco indicated to the authors in various interviews in March and April 2003 that such high percentage reduction had not been achieved with their patients in the same four-month period. Nonetheless, they added that calcium scores often began to fall dramatically if the patients continued for more time. The treatment time frame and conditions of patients seem key. More will be learned about this as additional studies occur.

7. Suggested retail price in correspondence from Nanobac Pharmaceuticals to physicians, February 26, 2004.

8. "Transfer Factor MycoPlus Physician Fact Sheet," http://www.advancedmedicallabs.com/shop/product.cfm?product__code=AM183 (accessed March 15, 2004).

9. N. Çíftçíoglu et al., "Inhibition of Nanobacteria by Antimicrobial Drugs as Measured by a Modified Microdilution Method," *Antimicrobial Agents and Chemotherapy* 46, no. 7 (July 2002): 2077–86, http://www.pubmedcentral.nih.gov/articlerender.fcgi?artid=127303 (accessed August 15, 2004).

10. Paul W. Ewald, *Plague Time: How Stealth Infections Cause Cancers, Heart Disease and Other Deadly Ailments* (New York: Anchor Books, 2002), pp. 232–33.

11. *The Sinatra Health Report*, the monthly subscription newsletter of Stephen Sinatra, M.D., F.A.C.C., June 2002.

CHAPTER 12: WHO PAYS?

1. Janelle Carter, "Health Care Spending Jumps 8.7 Percent," *Associated Press*, January 8, 2003, http://www.firstcoastnews.com/health/articles/2003-01-08/health_spending.asp (accessed March 11, 2004), reporting on the annual report of the Centers for Medicare and Medicaid; and "Survey: Health Insurance Premiums Up 14 Percent," *Houston Business Journal*, September 11, 2003, http://www.bizjournals.com/houston/stories/2003/09/08/daily37.html (accessed March 11, 2004).

2. Patient Directed Care Web site, http://www.patientdirectedcare.com (accessed January 23, 2004).

3. Interview with Alan Iezzi, October 16, 2002.

4. Joanna L. Krotz, "Check Out the Revolution in Health Care," bCentral, August 2003, http://www.bcentral.com/articles/krotz/140.asp (accessed April 1, 2004).

5. Keates, "The Holistic Hospital," *Wall Street Journal,* March 28, 2003: W1.

6. Interview with Alan Iezzi, October 16, 2002.

7. A list of insurers was provided in an e-mail to the authors from NanobacLabs, January 15, 2003, and updated in a fax, September 12, 2003.

MILESTONES

1. R. L. Folk, "SEM Imaging of Bacteria and Nannobacteria in Carbonate Sediments and Rocks," *Journal of Sedimentary Petrology* 63 (1993): 990–99.

2. E. Olavi Kajander, "Culture and Detection Method for Sterile-Filterable Autonomously Replicating Biological Particles," U.S. Patent no. 5,135,851, 16 pp., 1992.

3. E. O. Kajander, E. Tahvanainen, I. Kuronen, and N. Çiftçioğlu, "Comparison of Staphylococci and Novel Bacteria-like Particles from Blood," abstract, 7th International Symposium on Staphylococci and Staphylococcal Infections, June 29–July 3, 1992, Stockholm, Abstract book, p. 79, 1992. Also, K. Ackerman, Kuronen, and Kajander, "Scanning Electron Microscopy of Nanobacteria—Novel Biofilm Producing Organisms in Blood," *Scanning* 15, no. III (1993).

4. McKay et al., "Search for Past Life on Mars: Possible Relic Biogenic Activity in Martian Meteorite ALH 84001," *Science* 273 (August 16, 1996): 924–30.

5. N. Çiftçioğlu et al., "A New Potential Threat in Antigen and Antibody Products: Nanobacteria," in *Vaccines* 97, eds. Brown et al. (Cold Spring Harbor, NY: Cold Spring Harbor Laboratory Press, 1997), 99–103.

6. K. K. Åkerman, J. T. Kuikka, N. Çiftçioğlu, J. Parkkinen, K. A. Bergström, I. Kuronen, and E. O. Kajander, "Radiolabeling and In Vivo Distribution of Nanobacteria in Rabbit," *Proceedings SPIE* 3111 (1997): 436–42.

7. Kajander and N. Çiftçioğlu, "Nanobacteria: An Alternative Mechanism for Pathogenic Intra- and Extracellular Mineralisation and Stone Formation," *Proceedings of the National Academy of Sciences (PNAS)* USA 95, no. 14 (1998): 8274–79.

8. N. Çiftçioğlu, V. Çiftçioğlu, H. Vali, E. Turcott, and E. O. Kajander, "Sedimentary Rocks in our Mouth: Dental Pulp Stones Made by Nanobacteria," *Proceedings SPIE* 3441 (1998): 130–35.

9. E. Garcia-Cuerpo et al., "Nanobacteria. Un Modelo de Neo-litogenesis Experimental," *Arch Esp Urol* 53, no. 4 (2000): 291–303.

10. J. T. Hjelle et al., "Endotoxin and Nanobacteria in Polycystic Kidney Disease," *Kidney International* 57 (2000): 2360–74.

11. Kajander, N. Çiftçioğlu, and Aho, "Detection of Nanobacteria in Viral Vaccines," *Proceedings of the American Society for Microbiology*, 101st General Meeting, Orlando, FL, May 20–24, 2001, abstract Y-3, p. 736. Michael Le Page, "The Tiny Villains Lurking in Vaccines," *New Scientist* 170, no. 2293 (June 3, 2001): 12.

12. Rasmussen et al., "Electron Microscope and Immunological Evidence of Nanobacteria-like Structures," *J Am Coll Cardiol* 39, no. 5 (March 6, 2002): Supplement A.

13. N. Çiftçioğlu, "Risk for Nanobacteria in Gamma Globulin Preparations," 102nd General Meeting of the American Society for Microbiology.

14. Y. Li, Y. Wen, Z. Yang, H. Wei, W. Liu, A. Tan, X. Wu, Q. Wang, S. Huang, E. O. Kajander, and N. Çiftçioğlu, "Culture and Identification of Nanobacteria in Bile" [in Chinese, abstract PubMed PMID: 12609067], *Zhonghua Yi Xue Za Zhi* 82, no. 22 (November 25, 2002): 1557–60.

15. Martin Kerner, Heinz Hohenberg, Siegmund Ertl, Marcus Reckermann, and Alejandro Spitzy, "Self-organization of Dissolved Organic Matter to Micelle-like Microparticles in River Water," *Nature* 422 (March 13, 2003): 150–54.

16. Maniscalco, "Shouldering the Risk Burden," *Circulation* (March 25, 2003); B. S. Maniscalco and K. A. Taylor, "Calcification in Coronary Artery Disease Can Be Reversed by EDTA–Tetracycline Long-Term Chemotherapy," *Pathophysiology* DOI:10.1016/j.pathophys.2004.06.001 (accepted June 3, 2004).

17. Kajander et al., "The Pathogenesis Of Vascular Calcification," Poster session, Tampere, Finland, February 21, 2003.

18. Sedivy and Battistutti, "Nanobacteria Promote Crystallization of Psammoma Bodies in Ovarian Cancer," *APMIS* 111 (2003): 951–54.

19. Khullar et al., "Morphological and Immunological Characteristics of Nano-bacteria from Human Renal Stones of a North Indian Population," *Urol Res* 32, no. 3 (June 2004): 190–95.

20. E-mail communication from Katja M. Aho to the authors, March 9, 2004.

21. Jelic et al., "Nanobacteria-caused Mitral Valve Calciphylaxis in a Man with Diabetic Renal Failure," *South Med J* 97, no. 2 (February 2004): 194–98.

22. Lieske et al., "Detection and Propagation of Calcified Nanostructures from Human Aneurysms," *J Am Coll Cardiol Abstract Book*, 2004: 1059–13: 13 A. And Virginia M. Miller et al., "Evidence of Nanobacterial-like Structures in Human Calcified Arteries and Cardiac Valves," *Am J Physiol Heart Circ Physiol* 287, no. 3 (September 2004): H1115–24.

23. "Nanobac Life Sciences Announces Positive Results of Its Nanobacterial Anti-body Test for Coronary Artery Disease. Simple Blood Test Shows Correlation with Coronary Artery Calcification," Press Release, Nanobac Life Sciences, April 27, 2004, http://www.nanobaclabs.com/NewsRoom/PressReleases/Article.aspx?shortname=News_2004-04-27 (accessed April 27, 2004).

24. X. J. Wang, W. Liu , Z. L. Yang, H. Wei, Y. Wen, and Y. G. Li, "The Detection of Nanobacteria Infection in Serum of Healthy Chinese People" [in Chinese, abstract PubMed PMID: 15231124], *Zhonghua Liu Xing Bing Xue Za Zhi* 25, no. 6 (June 2004): 492–94.

GLOSSARY

1. Uffe Ravnskov, "The Cholesterol Myths: Exposing the Fallacy that Saturated Fat and Cholesterol Cause Heart Disease," NewTrends Publishing, Inc., 2000. Excerpts found at http://www.heart-disease-bypass-surgery.com/data/articles/36.htm#references (accessed April 5, 2004).

2. "CRP Improves Cardiovascular Risk Prediction in Metabolic Syndrome, Circulation," *Journal of the American Heart Association*, January 1, 2003,

   http://www.americanheart.org/presenter.jhtml?identifier=3007985 (accessed
   April 3, 2004).

3. "Computer Imaging/Tomography," American Heart Association, http://www
   .americanheart.org/presenter.jhtml?identifier=4554#ct (accessed April 3,
   2004).

4. "Fibrinogen," Medline Plus, National Library of Medicine, November 25,
   2001, http://www.nlm.nih.gov/medlineplus/ency/article/003650.htm (accessed
   April 5, 2004).

5. "What Is High Blood Pressure?" National Heart, Lung, and Blood Institute,
   NIH, http://www.nhlbi.nih.gov/hbp/hbp/whathbp.htm (accessed April 5,
   2004).

6. "Lipids," Springfield Technical Community College, http://distance.stcc
   .edu/AandP/AP/AP1pages/epitissmol/lipids.htm (accessed April 25, 2004).

7. "MRI," Medline Plus, National Library of Medicine, November 28, 2001,
   http://www.nlm.nih.gov/medlineplus/ency/article/003335.htm (accessed April
   4, 2004).

8. M. L. Knudtson, D. G. Wyse, P. D. Galbraith, et al., "Chelation Therapy for
   Ischemic Heart Disease: A Randomized Controlled Trial," *JAMA* 287 (2002):
   481–86, abstract, http://www.ncbi.nlm.nih.gov/entrez/query.fcgi?cmd=Retri
   eve&db=PubMed&list_uids=11798370&dopt=Abstract (accessed April 5,
   2004).

9. "ESR," Medline Plus, National Library of Medicine, November 23, 2001,
   http://www.nlm.nih.gov/medlineplus/ency/article/003638.htm (accessed April
   5, 2004).

10. "Drug to Lower Cholesterol Also Slows Calcium Buildup in Arteries,"
    Journal Report, American Heart Association, Feruary 8, 2002, http://www
    .Americanheart.org/presenter.jhtml;jsessionid=2RZC0OMO5WABBWFZ
    OAGSCZQ?identifier=3004052 (accessed April 3, 2004).

WHO'S WHO IN THE WORLD OF CALCIFICATION AND NANOBACTERIA

1. R. Y. Morita, "Bioavailability of Energy and Starvation Survival in Nature,"
   Canadian Journal of Microbiology 34 (1988): 436–41.

2. R. Y. Morita, *Bacteria in Oligotrophic Environments: Starvation-Survival Life
   Styles* (Dordrecht, Netherlands: Kluwer Academic Publishers, 1997).

About the Authors

D ouglas Mulhall's previous book, *Our Molecular Future*, coresearched by Katja Hansen, was selected by *New Scientist* magazine for its "must-read" list, featured in best-seller lists of Barnes and Noble and Amazon.com, and chosen as a finalist in the Independent Publishers Book Award Science category. It has been praised by numerous other organizations such as the Foresight Institute and the Association of College and Research Libraries, who chose it as an Outstanding Academic Title. Libraries around the world now carry the book, which is described further at www.OurMolecularFuture.com.

Mulhall's journalistic and Hansen's biological engineering backgrounds are supported by years of experience managing the disease prevention and environmental science programs of international scientific research institutes. They have cofounded and managed European and South American organizations devoted to research and communications. Their experience with preventing microbiological infections comes from pioneering water purification technologies in collaboration with multinational chemical companies and multilateral government agencies. The systems are now being replicated on three continents.

Other works of Mulhall and Hansen show how technology convergence is transforming our lives in everything from water recycling to world exposi-tions. Their articles are published by *Financial Times; Newsday; National Post; The Futurist; Futures Research Quarterly; Frankfurter Allgemeine Zeitung; Water, Environment and Technology*; the National Research Council; and the Center for Responsible Nanotechnology, to mention a few.

Index

See the glossary beginning on page 155 for definitions of technical terms. Names of researchers mentioned in the main body of the book are included in this index. However, see also "Milestones" beginning on page 147 and "Who's Who in the World of Calcification and Nanobacteria" beginning on page 165 for other individuals associated with the field.

microscopy, *continued*
   nanobacteria and, 26–29, 33–34, 61
   nanobacteria photographs, 42f–43f
microvascular disease. *See* vascular system disorders
middle ear ossification, 4f
Miller-Hjelle, Marcia, 52, 149, 168
mineralization. *See* biomineralization; calcification; crystallization
minerals, 94
monoclonal antibodies, 33–34, 148
MRI. *See* magnetic resonance imaging (MRI)
multiple sclerosis (MS), 4f, 8f, 10, 184n9
mycobacteria, 26
mycoplasmas, 26–30, 73f

N

nannobacteria, 38, 41–43, 169–70
nanoarchaeae, 40, 169–70
Nanoarchaeum equitans, 39–40, 42
Nanobac Life Sciences, 97, 149–50, 206n1, 211n6
Nanobac Oy, 31, 89, 149, 169, 204n3
Nanobac Pharmaceuticals, Inc., 150
nanobacteria
   atherosclerosis and, 143, 173–75, 199n13
   bisphosphonates and, 120
   cell infiltration and, 43f
   characteristics, 32–33, 42f, 48–50, 55f
   clarifying terminology of, 141
   clumping of, 28, 32, 99
   cross-reactivity to bacteria, 54
   culture contamination, 29–33
   defined, xi–xii, 40–43
   detection methods, 28–30, 47–48, 54–57, 127–28, 204n3
   diagnostic methods, 79–81
   discovery, 25–26, 84, 92
   environmental sources for, 63–64
   genetics, 33–34
   infection process, 34–35, 55–57, 75–76
   in vitro, 25, 126, 199n13
   in vivo, 126, 199n13
   Koch's Postulates and, 61–62
   life cycle of, 40–44
   nutritional supplements and, 90–91
   patenting of, 28–29
   research support of, 37–38
   resistance to drugs, 140
   size of, 35f, 43–44, 48–49
   symbiotic processes in, 31–32
   timeline and milestones, 147–50
   transfer factor, 127–28

   treatment for, 34, 62, 83–84
   treatment risks and, 124–25
   See also antibodies; blood nanobacteria
Nanobacterium sanguineum, 28–30, 50f, 111, 145
   See also blood nanobacteria; human nanobacteria; nanobacteria
nanobes, xi–xii, 39, 56–57, 59, 141, 169–70, 193n25
nanobiotics, 84, 197n67
   ampicillin and, 84
   bisphosphonates and, 84
   case histories, 106–10
   chelation therapy and, 95–97
   citrate and, 84
   clinical trials, 112–17
   commercial development of, 91–92, 127–28, 206n1
   costs of, 127, 135
   criticism of, 125–29, 169
   as cure, 127–28, 139–40
   defined, xi–xii
   EDTA and, 84
   ethics and, 128–29
   healthcare costs and, 135–36
   heart disease and, 85–86
   ingredients, 84, 94
   nutritional supplements and, 90–91, 97–100
   as panacea, 121, 125
   patenting, 84
   patient compliance and, 98–100
   preventative healthcare and, 134
   side effects, 116, 123f
   therapy developments, 89–90, 145–46
   treatment risks, 121–25
   See also nutritional supplements
nanofiltration, 139
NASA. *See* U.S. National Aeronautics and Space Administration (NASA)
National Academy of Sciences (NAS), 40, 52
Nature, 45
naturopathy, 86–87
   See also alternative therapies
NIH. *See* U.S. National Institutes of Health (NIH)
nitrofurantoin, 84
nucleic acids, 47–50
   See also deoxyribonucleic acid (DNA); ribonucleic acid (RNA)
nutraceuticals. *See* nanobiotics; nutritional supplements
nutritional supplements
   calcification and, 9
   nanobiotics and, xi–xii, 90–91